"This work by Dr. Kalant gives a welcome return to objectivity. [It] gives a masterly and succinct review of the knowledge to date. To the medical man it will afford a convenient and readable form of enlightenment on this very controversial subject. Students, too, will learn from it a great deal which may stand them in good stead, as much personally as it will professionally. But, above all, this should be obligatory reading for all those editors, radio and television producers, correspondents and moral arbiters who are so impatient to express themselves without paying sufficient attention to the facts that are available." Roy Goulding, *Proceedings of the Royal Society of Medicine*, on the first edition.

ORIANA JOSSEAU KALANT has degrees in biochemistry and in physiology. She has served as a member of the teaching staff of the department of physiology in the University of Chile, and as a research associate in the department of pharmacology in the University of Toronto. Since 1965 Dr. Kalant has been in the Research Division of the Addiction Research Foundation, Toronto.

THE AMPHETAMINES: TOXICITY AND ADDICTION

PUBLICATIONS
OF THE ADDICTION RESEARCH FOUNDATION

By the same author, with Harold Kalant, *Drugs, Society and
Personal Choice* (General Publishing, Don Mills, Ontario, 1971).

THE AMPHETAMINES
Toxicity and Addiction

ORIANA JOSSEAU KALANT, PH.D.

SECOND EDITION

Brookside Monograph of the Addiction Research Foundation No. 5

PUBLISHED FOR THE ADDICTION RESEARCH FOUNDATION

BY UNIVERSITY OF TORONTO PRESS

AND CHARLES C THOMAS

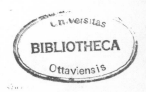

First edition
© UNIVERSITY OF TORONTO PRESS 1966

Second edition
© UNIVERSITY OF TORONTO PRESS 1973
Toronto and Buffalo

Printed in Canada

ISBN 0-8020-1835-1

Published and distributed in the U.S.A. by

CHARLES C THOMAS · PUBLISHER

Bannerstone House
301–327 East Lawrence Avenue, Springfield, Illinois, U.S.A.

Natchez Plantation House
735 North Atlantic Boulevard, Fort Lauderdale, Florida, U.S.A.

Foreword

FOR SEVERAL DECADES the amphetamines and substances related to them have been well known and used widely in clinical medicine. If pharmacologically and chemically related substances are included they have been used much more widely without medical supervision. Those who have prescribed the drugs, those concerned with their control, those who have taken them occasionally, or those who have become dependent on their use have assessed their value in rather different ways. A great deal of conflicting evidence has been reviewed by numerous writers in the past, but often has served only to reinforce the reviewers' preconceptions.

The Government of the Province of Ontario had reason to question the use or misuse of amphetamines and related compounds by certain occupational groups and sought advice on the hazard to the individual and to the public which might be incurred. A survey of existing knowledge of at least some aspects of the problem appeared desirable, and this was undertaken by the author of this book.

Of the various hazards associated with the misuse of these drugs, the most controversial and also potentially the most serious appeared to be that of addiction. The seriousness had been suggested some years earlier by Dr. P. H. Connell, who drew attention to the schizophrenia-like reaction which could be produced by excessive use of amphetamines. The controversy continued, however, because of several unresolved problems. One problem related to the lack of universal agreement on the concepts of drug addiction, habituation, and dependence. Another was the lack of suitable statistics to permit a reasonable conclusion about the frequency with which amphetamine misuse and its consequences occur in different parts of the world. Yet another was the constant intrusion of moral judgments and preconceptions into a matter which called for a clear, scientifically valid examination.

All of these problems have been tackled in the present study. As I have had the pleasure of working with and being associated with Dr. Oriana Josseau Kalant for many years, it was with no great surprise, but at the same time with admiration, that I observed her painstaking approach to the survey. It became apparent that this was no cursory review, but a detailed and careful analysis of the evidence respecting the amphetamines.

Finally, a rational approach to problems of addiction must take some cognizance of the degree of social acceptance and possible value of the substance under discussion. This approach has been emphasized in the present work, in respect to the amphetamines.

I think the present monograph will form a firm base for future investigations in this field. It provides an excellent example of the type of critical and unbiased approach which is essential for effective study of drugs and naturally occurring substances which may have addictive properties.

E. A. SELLERS, M.D., PH.D.,
Professor and Head of the
Department of Pharmacology,
Associate Dean of Medicine,
University of Toronto

Preface

A SURVEY OF THE LITERATURE on drugs of the amphetamine group was undertaken at the request of the Department of Health of the Government of Ontario. The original purpose of the survey was to find answers to these four questions.

1. What are the physiological and psychological effects of the amphetamines in the normal individual?

2. When can the drugs be used with advantage by a normal individual?

3. What are the dangers from their use, either to the individual or to society?

4. What are the addicting properties of the drugs?

The survey revealed that up to the end of 1961 there were approximately 2,200 articles concerning the amphetamines, which could be distributed roughly under the following headings: physiological effects, 1,100 references; effects on behavior, 220 references; medical uses, 420 references; psychiatric uses, 210 references; toxic and other untoward effects, 200 references; others, 50 references. Papers on the amphetamines have continued to appear at the rate of over 100 titles per year.

Thorough but outdated review articles on the pharmacology of the amphetamines are those of the Council on Pharmacy and Chemistry (United States) (47), Ivy and Krasno (100), and Ivy and Goetzl (101). Bett, Howells, and Macdonald (26) and Leake (116) have, within the past 10 years, published monographs with special emphasis on the clinical uses of the drugs. Wikler (197) has reviewed and discussed the biochemical, neurophysiological, and psychological mechanisms of amphetamine action. The effects of these drugs on human behavior and performance have recently been reviewed by Trouton and Eysenck (179) and by Weiss and Laties (190). In 1958 Connell (42) published a monograph entitled *Amphetamine Psychosis* which included 42 original cases of the condition and a thorough discussion of its characteristics. The most comprehensive study on the amphetamines was published in 1954 by Bonhoff and Lewrenz (29) under the title *Ueber Weckamine*. This work includes a review of 578 references and deals with the physiological and psychological effects of the drugs, their toxic manifestations, and amphetamine psychosis and amphetamine addiction, with descriptions of original clinical material. The most recent work dealing with the untoward effects of the amphetamines in man, and especially with the side effects of amphetamine therapy, was published by Welsh (191) in 1962.

Perusal of these reviews and monographs made it evident that the effects of amphetamines on human performance had been reviewed and discussed in at least two recent and comprehensive articles. The dangers involved in the use of amphetamines and the addicting properties of the drugs, on the other hand, had not been comprehensively reviewed since 1954 (29) and because that work was published in German it might be inaccessible to many readers. In addition, the literature concerning some of the toxic effects of the amphetamines and their habit-forming or addictive liabilities was highly controversial. For these reasons it was decided to focus this survey on the literature concerning the toxicity of amphetamines in man and the important but difficult problem of the characteristics of amphetamine abuse. This monograph attempts to answer the questions of what the dangers of amphetamine use are to the individual and to society and of whether or not they can be considered drugs of addiction.

This project was undertaken on the initiative of Professor E. A. Sellers, Head of the Department of Pharmacology of the University of Toronto. The author is greatly indebted to him for the opportunity to prepare this review. Dr. R. A. Hickie assisted in the gathering of references. The author is particularly grateful to Professor H. Kalant for his extensive and valuable discussions and suggestions throughout the course of the study and for detailed editorial review of the manuscript. Thanks are also due to Mr. R. E. Popham and Dr. R. J. Gibbins of the Alcoholism and Drug Addiction Research Foundation for their critical reading of the manuscript.

Preface to Second Edition

SINCE THE PUBLICATION of the first edition of this monograph in 1966 the developments surrounding the use of amphetamines and related drugs have been swift and dramatic, culminating, as this is being written, in the announcement by the government of Canada of close restrictions on the availability of these drugs for therapeutic purposes.

During the 1960s there occurred an explosive increase in the non-medical use of amphetamines, especially in North America and in some parts of Europe. This was part of the more general increase in the consumption of a variety of psychoactive drugs, but because of the nature of their effects and the pattern of use the amphetamines acquired a significance all their own. This newer pattern differed from that originally described in the monograph in a number of important respects. As a result, it acquired even a name of its own, the "speed" problem.

Many investigators have assumed that this is a totally new problem, unrelated to that described earlier. A critical examination reveals, however, that this differentiation is not justified on scientific grounds, and that the two aspects of the same problem continue to coexist. For this reason it was considered unnecessary to modify the text of the original version of this monograph, but highly desirable to add new sections dealing with the recent developments. This has been done by including three major appendices.

The author is most thankful to Dr. R. J. Gibbins for making available data on Toronto "speed" users, which are included in Appendix B, and to Mrs. C. Cox and Dr. R. G. Smart and the editors of the *Canadian Medical Association Journal* for permission to reprint the review as Appendix C. The dedicated and thorough cooperation of Mr. E. Polacsek and of Mrs. Lydia Vegers in the collection of references is highly appreciated. To Professor Harold

Kalant I am greatly indebted for help in many aspects of the preparation of this work, but most particularly for assisting me to keep the main objective in proper perspective.

March 1972   O.J.K.

Contents

List of Tables

THE AMPHETAMINES: TOXICITY AND ADDICTION

I. Introduction

THE TOXIC EFFECTS OF THE AMPHETAMINES which will be considered in this review, and the features which underlie their abuse and their addictive potential, are quantitative exaggerations of the same actions for which the drugs, in smaller doses, are beneficially employed. Before examining the undesirable effects, therefore, it is worth recalling what these drugs are and what characteristic pharmacological and therapeutic effects they produce.

The amphetamines are related both chemically and pharmacologically to a larger group of compounds generally known as pressor or sympathomimetic amines, such as epinephrine and ephedrine. Although they share with these compounds a frank sympathomimetic effect, the amphetamines have a proportionally greater stimulating effect on the central nervous system. In this respect they are also related to a newer group of drugs including phenmetrazine and diethylpropion, with which they share, in particular, a marked anorexigenic effect. The chemical similarity of all these substances is illustrated by their structural formulae (Figure 1).

For the purposes of this review the term amphetamines has been used to refer to racemic amphetamine, the dextrorotatory isomer *d*-amphetamine, and methamphetamine. Phenmetrazine and diethylpropion are usually considered amphetamine-like substances because though not phenylisopropyl amines they show both an obvious structural resemblance and very similar pharmacological effects to those of the amphetamines proper. The amphetamines have been available for pharmaceutical purposes as the free bases and as various salts, the most common of which are amphetamine and *d*-amphetamine sulfate and methamphetamine hydrochloride. These drugs are on the market under a variety of trade names, both singly and in combination with other

3

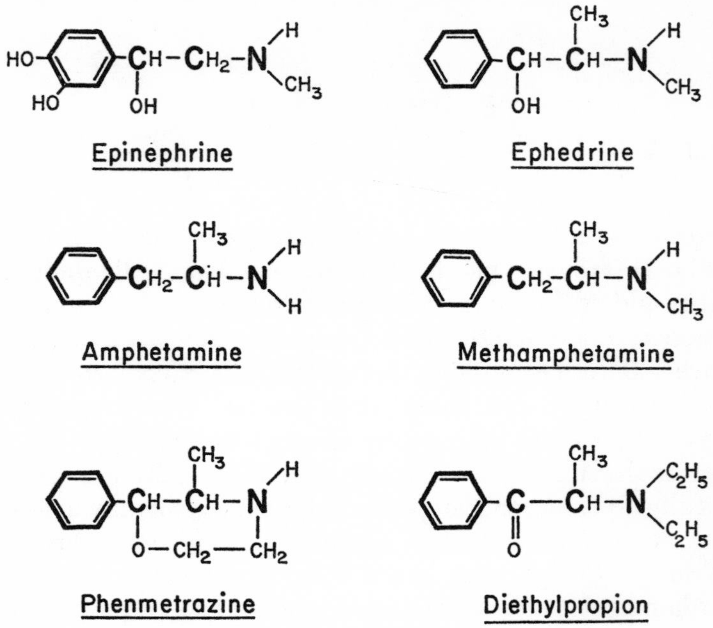

FIGURE 1

drugs such as barbiturates. Comprehensive lists of the amphetamine preparations currently available have been given by Leake (116), McCormick (127), and Welsh (191).

The peripheral effects of the amphetamines are generally those of the sympathomimetic amines. These include an increase in blood pressure as a result of an increase in both the heart rate and the peripheral vascular tone; pupillary dilatation; relaxation of the smooth muscle of the gastrointestinal tract, bronchioles, and urinary bladder; and secretion of sparse, thick saliva. The cardiovascular changes are clearly the most marked peripheral sympathomimetic effects of the amphetamines. When applied to mucosal surfaces the drugs produce local vasoconstriction; the use of amphetamine inhalers for the treatment of the common cold and hay fever was based on this action. However, widespread abuse of these devices led to their withdrawal from the market. Mydriasis, tachycardia, and hypertension are frequently noted as side effects of the drugs. The other sympathomimetic actions

4

are relatively minor, are not employed therapeutically, and give rise to side effects only when very large doses are taken.

In addition to these sympathomimetic effects many of the pressor amines also exert various stimulating effects on the central nervous system. The relative intensities of central and peripheral effects vary among the different drugs in this group. The amphetamines have the highest ratio of central to peripheral effect and are now used mainly for their central actions.

The most marked and consistent central effect is the production of a state of arousal or wakefulness, probably through a direct action upon the midbrain reticular formation. The arousal response is demonstrable both behaviorally and electroencephalographically and is accompanied by an increase in psychic and motor activity of all types. This effect is used therapeutically in the treatment of narcolepsy, and it also underlies the non-medical use of amphetamines for the improvement of performance and endurance by offsetting fatigue and sleepiness. The same effect, however, can be perceived as insomnia when it is not the primary objective. The effect on the reticular formation is probably responsible also for facilitation of sensory perception; it has been suggested that it is this effect carried to an extreme degree which explains the production of hallucinations in states of amphetamine intoxication.

Another prominent central action of amphetamines is the inhibition of appetite. There are conflicting views concerning the mechanism of production of anorexia. Some believe that this is a direct inhibitory effect upon hypothalamic appetite stimulating centres while others consider the effect secondary to cerebral stimulation. In either case the anorexigenic effect is the basis for what is perhaps the most frequent medical indication of the amphetamines at present, viz. the treatment of obesity. At the same time it constitutes another frequent side effect when the drugs are used for other purposes.

The central stimulatory effects are usually perceived subjectively as a sense of increased energy and self-confidence, and of faster and more efficient thought and decision-taking; it is usually accompanied by a feeling of well-being and even of euphoria. This effect is employed therapeutically in the treatment of some

5

types of depression, but it also is the basis for misuse of the drugs both by thrill-seekers and by people with inadequate personalities. In some cases, however, these same effects are perceived as an unpleasant increase in tension which can give rise to anxiety. When carried to extremes, they probably give rise to the flight of ideas, erratic behavior, and other mental disturbances that characterize severe toxic states.

This brief review will suffice to indicate the general nature of the toxic reactions which may result from misuse of the amphetamines and the close relation between therapeutic and toxic effects. In the chapters which follow, the various ill effects will be considered in detail not only from the point of view of fuller and more exact description but also with respect to their frequency and to their importance to the individual and to society.

II. Acute and Subacute
Amphetamine Intoxication

ACUTE INTOXICATION IN CHILDREN

IN VIEW OF THE WIDESPREAD USE of the amphetamines, reported cases of acute poisoning in children are rare. In all, 19 case reports have been found in the literature: 10 in the United States (94, 155, 65, 149, 108, 79, 136, and 127), 5 in the United Kingdom (114, 141, 164, 188, and 113), 2 in Argentina (182 and 71), and 2 in South Africa (148). Only 2 of these cases were fatal and in 1 of them it is questionable that death was exclusively due to amphetamine. These cases of amphetamine poisoning are accidental, of course, and have occurred mainly in young children who had access to bottles containing various amphetamine preparations.

The symptoms of amphetamine intoxication are the result of overstimulation of the sympathetic and central nervous systems. They appear between one and two hours after ingestion of the drug and increase in intensity over the next 24 to 48 hours, depending on dose and treatment. The severity of the picture depends on the dose, as well as on the susceptibility of the child to the drug. Ong (136) has classified the syndrome as mild, moderate, or severe on the basis of the symptoms listed in Table I.

General information concerning the cases reported in the literature is summarized in Table II, and the main symptoms are listed in Table III. The children ranged in age between 1 and 7.5 years, but the majority were between 2 and 3 years old. The estimated doses have ranged between 10 mg of amphetamine in the case of a 27-month-old boy (71) and 115 mg of d-amphetamine in a 32-month-old boy (141). These cases are too few to permit a

TABLE I

CLASSIFICATION OF SIGNS AND SYMPTOMS OF ACUTE AMPHETAMINE INTOXI-
CATION IN CHILDREN ACCORDING TO ONG (136)

Mild	Moderate	Severe
Restlessness	Confusion	Convulsions
Tremors	Delirium	Circulatory collapse
Insomnia	Hallucinations	Hyperpyrexia
Talkativeness	Panic states	Chest pain
Irritability	Profuse sweating	Coma and death
Tachycardia		
Flushing of the skin		
Increased sweating		
Mydriasis		
Dryness of the mouth		
Glycosuria		
Hyperactive reflexes		
Analgesia		
Fever		

sound conclusion respecting the relation of dose and severity of intoxication. For example, a 3-year-old boy who took an estimated 40 mg of d-amphetamine died 10.5 hours after the accident (148), whereas a 32-month-old boy who took 115 mg of d-amphetamine recovered after 5 days of treatment (141). In this respect wide individual variation in response to the drug cannot be excluded as a possible explanation, but it is probable that other factors, such as time elapsed between ingestion of the drug and the beginning of therapy and the type of treatment given, may have had a bearing on the course of the syndrome. In the fatal case reported by Pretorius (148), for example, stomach lavage was not performed until 2.5 hours after ingestion of the drug when the symptoms of intoxication were already extremely severe, whereas in the case reported by Patuck (141) this was done 1 hour after the accident, although Patuck states that no remnants of tablets were found. Furthermore, sensory isolation was used in the latter case but not in the former.

As Table III shows, the most constant symptoms reported are mydriasis, tachycardia, motor excitation, and insomnia. Motor restlessness, obviously the most dramatic of the symptoms, was present in all instances, except in the fatal case reported by Hertzog, et al. (94), where the child was found in a state of collapse from which she did not recover. These symptoms are obviously exaggerations of the usual sympathomimetic and

TABLE II

REPORTED CASES OF AMPHETAMINE INTOXICATION IN CHILDREN

Author	Reference	Sex	Age	Drug*	Stated dose
Hertzog, *et al.* (1943) U.S.A.	94	F	12 mo.	dl-A SO₄ FeSO₄	40 mg unknown
Rosenbaum (1943) U.S.A.	155	F	20 mo.	dl-A SO₄	unknown
Vidal Freyre (1947) Argentina	182	M	25 mo.	dl-A SO₄	70–80 mg
Gerscovich (1948) Argentina	71	M	27 mo.	dl-A SO₄	10 mg
Langham (1950) U.K.	114	M	24 mo.	d-A SO₄	25 mg
Fletcher (1953) U.S.A.	65	M	24 mo.	d-A SO₄ phenobarbital	40–50 mg 60–75 mg
Pretorius (1953) S. Africa	148	M F	3 yr. 5 yr.	d-A SO₄ d-A SO₄	40 mg 40 mg
Rapp (1953) U.S.A.	149	F	22 mo.	d-A SO₄ (Spansules)	60 mg
Keiter & Arnold (1955) U.S.A.	108	F F F	16 mo. 18 mo. 24 mo.	d-A SO₄ d-A SO₄ d-A SO₄	unknown unknown 6–8 tablets
Patuck (1956) U.K.	141	M	32 mo.	d-A SO₄	115 mg
Shanson (1956) U.K.	164	M	7.5 yr.	dl-A (?)	unknown
Watts (1956) U.K.	188	M	28 mo.	dl-A SO₄ aspirin phenacetin	unknown
Gullat (1957) U.S.A.	79	M	21 mo.	meth-A HCl phenobarbital	70 mg 450 mg
Lancer (1961) U.K.	113	M	5 yr.	d-A SO₄	15 mg in 3 days
Ong (1962) U.S.A.	136	M	3 yr.	d-A SO₄	100 mg
McCormick (1962) U.S.A.	127	M	4 yr.	d-A SO₄ (Spansules)	75–90 mg

*d-A SO₄—d-amphetamine sulfate dl-A SO₄—amphetamine sulfate

meth-A—methamphetamine base dl-A—amphetamine base   meth-A HCl—methamphetamine hydrochloride

TABLE III

SYMPTOMS OF ACUTE AMPHETAMINE INTOXICATION IN CHILDREN

Author	Flushing	Sweating	Fever	Anuria	Dryness of mouth	Mydriasis	Tachycardia	Raised B.P.	Vomiting	Increased respirations	Tremor	Hyperactive reflexes	Motor excitation	Euphoria	Logorrhea	Insomnia	Fear	Panic	Confusion	Hallucinations	Delirium	Exhaustion	Circulatory collapse	Coma	Death	Duration
Hertzog, et al.						×	×		×	×			×			×							×	×	×	21 hr.
Rosenbaum						×	×		×				×			×										24 hr.
Vidal Freyre				×		×	×						×			×										36 hr.
Gerscovich			×	×		×	×						×			×										24 hr.
Langham	×					×	×			×			×			×	×		×							46 hr.
Fletcher	×					×	×		×	×		×	×		×	×	×		×		×					48 hr.
Pretorius			×			×	×						×	×	×	×					×					10.5 hr.
													×			×				×			×		×	48 hr.
Rapp	×												×			×							×			48 hr.
Keiter & Arnold											×		×			×										48 hr.
													×	×	×	×		×	×	×						24 hr.
													×		×	×		×		×						24 hr.
Patuck	×					×			×	×			×	×		×		×								5 days
Shanson						×	×						×		×	×			×	×						48 hr.
Watts							×						×		×	×			×							48 hr.
Gullat					×		×	×	×				×			×										3 days
Lancer	×		×			×				×			×		×	×				×						48 hr.
Ong	×					×	×					×	×		×	×						×	×		×	30 hr.
McCormick	×	×				×							×	×		×			×	×		×				10 hr.
TOTALS FOR 19 CASES	**6**	**1**	**3**	**2**	**1**	**12**	**12**	**1**	**4**	**5**	**1**	**2**	**18**	**3**	**7**	**15**	**3**	**3**	**5**	**5**	**2**	**2**	**2**	**1**	**2**	

central stimulatory effects produced by normal therapeutic doses of the drugs. They reach their peak a few hours after ingestion of the drugs and last in most cases between 24 and 48 hours, although such signs as ataxia and euphoria may persist for several days (65).

Treatment is symptomatic. Stomach lavage has been performed in most cases, but it appears that by the time the symptoms are marked enough to require medical attention, it is too late for this procedure to be effective. Since motor restlessness, or in most instances wild excitation, is the most prominent symptom, sedation is of paramount importance. For this purpose barbiturates, especially phenobarbital, have been used in almost every case, but when the intoxication is severe this does not appear to be effective enough. In fact, in two of the cases reviewed here the child took preparations containing a mixture of amphetamines and barbiturates (65 and 79), but the symptoms of amphetamine intoxication prevailed. Other measures used for this purpose have been the intramuscular administration of paraldehyde and of hypertonic $MgSO_4$ and the intravenous administration of chlorpromazine. Magnesium sulfate, first used by Vidal Freyre (182), was also used by Pretorius (148) and by Patuck (141) because of its depressant effect on the central nervous system, its curare-like action peripherally, and its ability to prevent cerebral edema and congestion.

In 1956 Hopkin and Jones (97) recommended the use of chlorpromazine in cases of amphetamine poisoning because according to them this tranquilizer has been shown to depress conduction of nerve impulses through the reticular activating system,* to block the effects of d-amphetamine on the reticular system of cats when given either before or after d-amphetamine administration, and to control the restlessness produced by an overdose of Adrenalin, the central action of which is also on the reticular system. In 1957 Gullat (79) reported dramatic results following the intravenous administration of chlorpromazine to a 21-month-old boy who had taken 70 mg of methamphetamine.

*Recent evidence (108a) indicates that chlorpromazine depresses the collateral afferent sensory input into the reticular formation, rather than conduction within the reticular activating system itself. However, this does not invalidate the basic concept of this treatment.

Hydration is also important, because the amphetamines are excreted unchanged in the urine. According to Beyer and Skinner (27) about 43 per cent of a 20–30 mg dose is excreted in the urine in the first 48 hours. In addition, the frequent occurrence of fever and sweating indicate the importance of an adequate fluid intake.

Chance (38) observed that the lethal dose of amphetamine for mice caged singly was 117 mg/kg, as opposed to 14 mg/kg for mice in groups of 10 per cage. A related observation by Patuck (141), in the case of a 32-month-old boy who had taken 115 mg d-amphetamine, was that every sensory stimulus appeared to aggravate the hyperactivity. Therefore, in addition to barbiturates and $MgSO_4$, Patuck employed sensory isolation as a therapeutic measure. The child was nursed in a darkened soundproof cubicle, in a cot with padded sides. No other author seems to have made use of this ingenious procedure.

Ong (136) has suggested that sedatives be used with caution because many commercial preparations of amphetamines contain barbiturates as well, and because of the depressive phase that sometimes follows the acute symptoms of amphetamine intoxication. He has also suggested the use of extracorporeal dialysis in cases with high blood levels of amphetamine, as well as anti-hypertensive measures and intravenous administration of urea if symptoms of cerebral edema appear.

The three case histories which follow are illustrative of moderate, severe, and fatal degrees of amphetamine intoxication in children.

Case Histories

CASE 1 (188). A 28-month-old boy ate an unknown number of Edrisal tablets, each containing 2.5 mg of amphetamine and 160 mg of aspirin and phenacetin respectively. The child was normally quiet and retiring but after this he became more and more active, although ataxic, and talkative. By night he was physically exhausted but unable to sleep. He talked all night long, sometimes incoherently, and vomited several times. When seen the next morning he was quiet for the first time. The pulse was 144 and the temperature normal. He was still ataxic but his speech was clear. He was given 8 mg of phenobarbital every 4 hours. He slept during the day, but was sick at intervals. The next day, after a good night's sleep, he was fully recovered.

12

CASE 2 (141). A 32-month-old boy accidentally took an estimated 115 mg of *d*-amphetamine sulfate. On his admission to hospital 1 hour later, stomach lavage produced no traces of the tablets. He was very restless with a pulse rate of 200 per minute. Over the following 5 hours, 2 ml of paraldehyde and 0.13 g of phenobarbital were given in divided doses, but his condition failed to improve. He became completely uncontrollable, rolling about and swinging his arms and legs continually. He was fully conscious and able to talk. His face was flushed, but his limbs and body were cold and clammy. The rectal temperature was 100° F, the heart rate 220 per minute, and the respirations very rapid. His eyes were staring, with widely dilated pupils which reacted normally to light. He was given 5 ml of 25% MgSO₄ intramuscularly and 65 mg of amobarbital at approximately 2-hour intervals and was nursed in a darkened soundproof cubicle in a cot with padded sides. Fourteen hours after the accident he was quieter, his pulse rate had decreased, and his general condition improved. During the second day in hospital he needed no further sedation or MgSO₄, but the hyperactivity persisted and he was confused and hallucinated. He remained irritable and excitable and when on the fourth day he was allowed to get up he had marked ataxia and euphoria. He was symptom free on the sixth day.

CASE 3 (148). A 3-year-old boy accidentally took an estimated 40 mg of *d*-amphetamine. One hour later he was restless and he vomited, urinated, and defecated in bed. His limbs flayed about uncontrollably but there were no convulsions. Despite 60 mg of phenobarbital and 100 mg of pentobarbital by rectum he was admitted to hospital 2.5 hours after the accident in a state of mania (extremely restless and unmanageable). Stomach lavage produced no remnants of the tablets. He was given 3 dr of paraldehyde by rectum and 10 ml of vitamin C intramuscularly and, 1 hour later, 180 mg of phenobarbital intramuscularly, but he continued agitated and confused. His skin was cold and clammy and his pupils were extremely dilated and non-reactive to light. Pulse and blood pressure were undetectable, but heart sounds were loud and clear. The heart rate was estimated at 200 per minute. Respirations were rapid and irregular but his chest was clear. Because of serious exhaustion and failure with previous therapy he was given 0.2 mg of scopolamine hydrobromide. This calmed him somewhat but another dose 1 hour later had no effect and he died 10.5 hours after the accident in complete exhaustion. The main findings at autopsy were marked edema of the brain and gross dilatation of the lateral and third ventricles with a pressure conus indicating internal hydrocephalus. Other findings were subendocardial bleeding, bilateral superficial pneumonia, closed hypoglottis and slight edema of the glottis, some edema of the spleen and kidneys, a fatty liver, and an enlarged thymus gland. Pretorius suggests that trepanation and

13

ventricular puncture might have relieved the internal hydrocephalus and pressure conus.

The other fatal case of "amphetamine sulfate poisoning," reported by Hertzog, *et al.*, in 1943 (94) is subject to question because the child ingested an undetermined number of ferrous sulfate tablets as well as an estimated 40 mg of amphetamine sulfate. The authors discarded the possibility of ferrous sulfate intoxication and concluded that death was the result of amphetamine poisoning. This does not seem to be justified because there was vomiting of brown material, hemorrhagic gastric mucosa with positive ferricyanide test, and rapid onset of coma, all of which are typical signs of massive ingestion of iron preparations, including ferrous sulfate (166).

The actual incidence of amphetamine poisoning in children in any given community cannot be estimated from the number of cases reported in the literature. Because only ten cases were reported in the United States over a period of approximately twenty-five years one might conclude that the problem is trivial. The fact is, rather, that the vast majority of cases have not been published. This is supported by Ong's statement (136) that 38 cases of amphetamine poisoning in children under 5 years of age were reported to the Boston Poison Information Center in 1959 alone. This is hardly surprising if it is considered that the production of amphetamines in the United States during 1958 was 75,000 pounds, or 3.5 billion tablets, or about 20 tablets for every man, woman, and child in the country (64). There must be many households in which enterprising children can find bottles of them to explore.

Figures for the city of Toronto between August, 1960, and August, 1963, were made available through the courtesy of Dr. R. J. Imrie and are summarized in Table IV. During that period 52 cases were seen at the Hospital for Sick Children; 11 of these required hospitalization for 2 or 3 days. The total number of cases of poisoning by ingestion in the same period was 4,594, so that poisoning by amphetamines accounted for 1.1 per cent of all cases of this type. Of the 52 children, 39 were between 2 and 3 years of age, a time when a child is very likely to test his environment by tasting it. The types and amounts of preparations taken

14

TABLE IV

ACUTE AMPHETAMINE POISONING IN CHILDREN SEEN AT THE
HOSPITAL FOR SICK CHILDREN IN TORONTO FROM AUGUST, 1960, TO
AUGUST, 1963, PATIENTS SEEN

Year	No. of cases	Age	
		Average	Range
1960–61	17	3 yr.	10 mo.–8 yr.
1961–62	18	2 yr., 5 mo.	1–6.5 yr.
1962–63	17	3 yr.	1.5–14 yr.

TABLE V

ACUTE AMPHETAMINE POISONING IN CHILDREN SEEN AT
THE HOSPITAL FOR SICK CHILDREN IN TORONTO FROM
AUGUST, 1960, TO AUGUST, 1963, PREPARATIONS INGESTED

Drugs*	Range of amounts
dl-A SO$_4$	20–60 mg
d-A SO$_4$	10–15 mg
Dexamyl tablets	
d-A SO$_4$, 5 mg	10–40 mg
amobarbital, 32 mg	64–256 mg
Dexamyl spansules	
d-A SO$_4$, 10 mg	230 mg
amobarbital, 65 mg	1495 mg
Meth-A HCl	unknown
Ambar extentabs # 2	
meth-A HCl, 15 mg	30 mg
phenobarbital, 65 mg	130 mg
Eskatrol	
d-A SO$_4$, 15 mg	15–30 mg
prochlorperazine, 7.5 mg	7.5–15 mg
Biphetamine	
equal parts of *d*-A and *dl*-A	7.5–125 mg

    *d-A SO$_4$—*d*-amphetamine sulfate
    dl-A—amphetamine base
    dl-A SO$_4$—amphetamine sulfate
    meth-A—methamphetamine base
    meth-A HCl—methamphetamine hydrochloride

are listed in Table V; it will be noticed that many of these are
commonly used for the treatment of obesity. It seems advisable
to caution mothers who use amphetamine preparations for reducing or other purposes about the potential dangers of these drugs.

This evidence indicates that the number of cases seen in one
year in a single hospital is about the same as the total number
reported in the world literature since the amphetamines came

into use over 30 years ago. It is obvious, therefore, that the frequency of case reports in the medical literature gives no indication of the true incidence of the condition. This conclusion most likely also applies to such other manifestations of adverse reactions to the amphetamines as addiction and toxic psychoses, to be discussed in later chapters.

Summary

Acute amphetamine poisoning in young children is accidental and is characterized by a dramatic picture of overstimulation of the sympathetic and central nervous systems. Mydriasis, tachycardia, insomnia, and extreme restlessness are the most frequent symptoms, and treatment is symptomatic. The incidence of this type of poisoning is far greater than the number of published reports would suggest.

ACUTE AND SUBACUTE INTOXICATION IN ADULTS

For the purpose of this review amphetamine intoxication, whether acute or subacute, is defined as an abnormal physical and/or mental state provoked by the intake of amphetamines for a period shorter than one month, and in most cases by a single large dose. Cases of this nature will be presented and examined separately from those due to prolonged abuse of amphetamines, because the latter present somewhat different problems. The presentation of the material in a comprehensive tabular form is difficult because a considerable number of cases were reported in groups rather than individually, and also because some of the reports dealing primarily with psychiatric conditions were not sufficiently explicit with respect to the physical condition of the patients. However, the major features of all the cases found in the literature that fitted this definition of acute and subacute amphetamine intoxication are summarized in Table VI.

Of a total of 54 cases, 26 were reported in the United Kingdom (4, 53, 186, 174, 144, 140, 77, 42, 21, 104, and 177), 14 in the United States (13, 56, 169, 70, 130, 49, 88, 90 & 92), 3 in Italy (143, 60 & 176), 3 in Germany (99 & 183), 2 in Puerto Rico (93),

TABLE VI

REPORTED CASES OF ACUTE AND SUBACUTE AMPHETAMINE INTOXICATION IN ADULTS

Author	Reference	Sex	Age	Drug*	Stated dose	Toxic psychotic symptoms	Other drugs taken simultaneously
Anderson & Scott (1936) U.K.	4	M	49	dl-A SO₄	30 mg		
Davies (1937) U.K.	53	M	26	dl-A SO₄	190 mg in 9 days		
Apfelberg (1938) U.S.A.	13	M	29	dl-A SO₄	140 mg		
Ehrich, et al. (1939) U.S.A.	56	M / M	67 / 27	dl-A SO₄ / dl-A SO₄	450 mg / 350 mg	x	alcohol
Issekutz (1939) Germany	99	F / M	23 / 26	meth-A HCl / meth-A HCl	60 mg / 200 mg		alcohol, coffee / alcohol, coffee
Smith (1939) U.S.A.	169	M	25	dl-A SO₄	30 mg in a few days		
Pous Chazaro (1941) Mexico	146	M	?	dl-A	part of one inhaler		
Pontrelli (1942) Italy	143	M	25	dl-A SO₄	?		
Carratalá & Calzetta (1943) Argentina	37	F	30	meth-A HCl	30 mg	x	
Gericke (1945) U.S.A.	70	M	36	dl-A SO₄	120 mg		
Monroe & Drell (1947) U.S.A.	130	M / M	30 / ?	dl-A / dl-A	93 mg in 36 hours / 250 mg	x / x	
Hernandez & Dalmau (1948) Puerto Rico	93	M / M	29 / 20	dl-A / dl-A	250 mg / 300 mg	x / x	
Curry (1949) U.S.A.	49	M	23	dl-A	250 mg		
Hart (1949) U.S.A.	88	F	?	dl-A	2250 mg in 2 weeks		

TABLE VI (cont.)

Author	Reference	Sex	Age	Drug*	Stated dose	Toxic psychotic symptoms	Other drugs taken simultaneously
Harvey, et al. (1949) U.S.A.	90	M	35	dl-A	250–500 mg	x	alcohol
Wallis, et al. (1949) U.K.	186	M	29	dl-A SO₄	55 mg	x	
Temkin (1953) U.K.	174	F	41	d-A SO₄	5 mg		
Herman & Nagler (1954) U.S.A.	92	M	23	dl-A	1 dose	x	
		M	23	dl-A	250 mg	x	
		M	32	dl-A	750 mg in 3 days	x	
		M	33	dl-A	? for 3 days		
Ruiz Ogara (1954) Spain	156	F	30	dl-A SO₄	10 mg I.V.	x	
Fedeli & Lumia (1955) Italy	60	M	33	meth-A HCl dl-A SO₄	250 mg		
Martimor, et al. (1955) France	120	M	29	dl-A SO₄	50 tablets	x	alcohol
Poteliakhoff & Roughton (1956) U.K.	144	M	42	dl-A	325 mg		
		M	28	dl-A	325 mg		coffee
Pathy (1957) U.K.	140	F	20	d-A SO₄	630 mg		
Greenwood & Peachey (1957) U.K.	77	M	23	dl-A	part of one inhaler	x	
		F	32	dl-A SO₄	200 mg		
		M	32	dl-A	487 mg		alcohol
Tolentino & D'Avossa (1957) Italy	176	M	30	dl-A SO₄	8-10 tablets in 2 days	x	alcohol

TABLE VI (concld.)

Author	Reference	Sex	Age	Drug*	Stated dose	Toxic psychotic symptoms	Other drugs taken simultaneously
Connell (1958) U.K.	42	M	23	dl-A	325 mg (?)	x	
		M	34	meth-A HCl	60 mg I.V. + 60 mg I.M.	x	
		M	33	meth-A	250 mg	x	
		F	23	dl-A	325 mg (?) in 3 days	x	
		F	29	dl-A	975 mg in 2 days	x	
		M	32	dl-A SO$_4$	75 mg	x	
		M	38	dl-A	325 mg ?	x	alcohol
		M	38	d-A SO$_4$	120 mg in 4 days	x	alcohol
		M	31	dl-A	325 mg } in 2–3 days	x	
				dl-A SO$_4$	50 mg }		
		M	35	dl-A	250–300 mg in 5–6 days	x	
		F	39	dl-A	325 mg in 4 days	x	
		M	31	dl-A	325 mg in 6 hours	x	
		M	20	dl-A	975 mg in 2 days	x	
Vill (1959) Germany	183	F	?	meth-A HCl	240–300 mg		
Ayache (1960) Morocco	16	F	24	d-A tartrate	?	x	caffeine, strychnine
Beamish & Kiloh (1960) U.K.	21	F	19	d-A SO$_4$ amobarbital	250 mg 1600 mg	x	
Bernheim & Cox (1960) Switzerland	24	M	25	dl-A SO$_4$ meth-A HCl	105 mg		coffee
Jordan & Hampson (1960) U.K.	104	F	25	dl-A SO$_4$	310 mg		
Tonks & Livingston (1963) U.K.	177	F	31	d-A; l-A	12.5 mg		phenelzine

*d-A SO$_4$—d-amphetamine sulfate   meth-A—methamphetamine base
dl-A—amphetamine base   meth-A HCl—methamphetamine hydrochloride
dl-A SO$_4$—amphetamine sulfate

and one each in Mexico (146), Argentina (37), Spain (156), France (120), Morocco (16), and Switzerland (24). Thirty-nine of these patients were men and 15 women, and their ages ranged from 19 to 67 years. The circumstances leading up to these intoxications were varied, although in at least 13 cases they were not reported. In only 5 of the remaining cases were amphetamines taken on medical prescription (174, 156, 16, and 177), the rest being instances of self-administration for various reasons such as to combat fatigue, improve intellectual or physical performance, treat common colds, or relieve depression. In 5 instances (37, 70, 93, and 183) there was suicidal intent.

The most commonly used drugs (39 of the 54 cases) were amphetamine base and amphetamine sulfate. Amphetamine base was widely available until recently, in the form of inhalers. In most cases, however, the drug was not taken by inhalation, but orally. The crudest technique consisted of chewing the strips of paper impregnated with amphetamine base, but since this caused irritation of the buccal mucosa more refined techniques were developed such as wrapping the strips in paper and swallowing them whole or dissolving the contents of the strips in coffee or alcoholic drinks (130). The types of drugs used and the methods of administration will be discussed more fully in chapter iv.

Table VI shows that the doses of amphetamines capable of producing a toxic state vary widely, from 5 to 630 mg in the case of *d*-amphetamine, although the 630-mg dose was taken in the form of a prolonged-release preparation. In most cases the dose was many times the therapeutic one.

The clinical picture of acute amphetamine poisoning in adults is basically the same as that observed in children; that is, it is characterized by signs of overstimulation of the sympathetic and central nervous systems. The most striking difference, however, is the high incidence in adults of psychotic reactions accompanied by relatively mild physical symptoms. Table VI shows that 30 of the 54 cases had psychotic symptoms consisting mainly of auditory and visual hallucinations and of delusions of persecution.

The six case histories given below were chosen as representative of the clinical picture found in acute amphetamine poisoning in adults.

20

Case Histories

CASE 1. In 1953 Temkin (174) reported the case of a healthy 41-year-old woman who was given 5 mg of *d*-amphetamine sulfate before meals because of mild depression and fatigue. Ten minutes after taking the first dose she complained of a feeling of impending death, frontal headache, giddiness, palpitation, and retrosternal discomfort. She was pale, cold, and clammy. Her temperature was subnormal and her pulse rate 90 per minute. She was given phenobarbital and put to bed. Seven hours later she was still clammy, her headache was now occipital and frontal, pulse rate 100, and blood pressure 110/75. Although the patient was rational she felt "miles away." The next day the patient was well except for a feeling of weakness. A subsequent test dose of 2.5 mg of *d*-amphetamine sulfate produced a similar but much less severe reaction.

CASE 2. Ruiz Ogara (156) reported the case of a 30-year-old widow with a reactive anxiety depression who was given 10 mg of amphetamine sulfate (Centramina) intravenously for exploratory purposes. After a few minutes the patient began to scream that she was being watched, and that the doctor wanted to kill her on orders from the Church. She was suspicious and hyperactive, but lucid. Later she developed visual and auditory hallucinations and vivid phantasies. These acute psychotic symptoms subsided after 2 days.

CASE 3. In 1955 Fedeli and Lumia (60) reported the case of a 33-year-old unemployed bar tender who ingested 250 mg of Stenamina (a mixture of methamphetamine hydrochloride and amphetamine sulfate). Half an hour later he had intense frontal headache, cold sweats, hyperexcitability, dryness of the mouth, palpitations, and abdominal pain. This was followed by loss of consciousness, violent tonic and clonic convulsions, especially of the upper limbs, drooling of saliva, pallor, firm fast pulse, and mydriasis. The blood pressure was 220/145. After sedation the symptoms subsided rapidly and the next day the patient was relatively normal, lucid, and calm, but there was moderate dysuria, lumbar pain, and bilateral subconjunctival hemorrhages. The patient was discharged recovered after 8 days.

CASE 4. Connell (42) describes the case of a 31-year-old man who ingested most of the contents of an amphetamine inhaler (325 mg) over a 6-hour period because he was feeling depressed and knew amphetamine "pepped you up." He became restless, began walking the streets, and spent the night in a park. He spent the next day looking for gold in the park and in the evening he thought he heard people talking about him and was sure that they were going to kill him. He also thought that cars and people were following him. Finally he climbed on a roof to get away and began to throw tiles at the crowds

21

he imagined in the streets below. He was taken by the police to the hospital. He was overactive, trembling, agitated, and terrified, but after 3 days he became calm and relaxed, and was no longer deluded or hallucinated. He had never had hallucinations or delusions of persecution before. He drank heavily but not continuously and was not an amphetamine addict.

CASE 5. Pathy (140) reported the case of a 20-year-old woman who became depressed and ingested 630 mg of d-amphetamine in the form of Spansule capsules. When admitted to hospital 9 hours later she was mildly excited but easily calmed by reassurance. The pulse rate was 110 per minute and the blood pressure 120/85. After treatment with $MgSO_4$ and barbiturates she slept well and the following morning she was symptom free. Since examination of the faeces 13.5 hours after admission revealed only one out of the 19,000 pellets ingested, it is probable that the patient absorbed most of the dose.

CASE 6. In 1945 Gericke (70) described the case of a 36-year-old physically normal soldier, undergoing psychotherapy because of periodic feelings of depression accompanied by heavy drinking, who was given 5 mg of amphetamine sulfate daily. During one of these periods of depression he decided to commit suicide by taking an overdose of amphetamine. It was estimated that he took 120 mg. He was admitted to hospital in a dazed condition. His pulse was 58, strong, and full, and he had an intense frontal headache. At 11:30 P.M. the right leg and arm became paralyzed and he had difficulty with breathing. Except for a rise in pulse rate to 80 per minute the condition remained unchanged until 4:00 A.M., when he vomited. The rectal temperature was 103.8° F. Despite caffeine and sodium benzoate and oxygen, the respiration became labored and his pulse rate rose to over 100. The patient's condition became steadily worse until he died at 4.55 A.M. Autopsy revealed that the immediate cause of death was subdural and subarachnoid hemorrhage of the parietal and occipital lobes.

These cases illustrate the wide degree of individual variation in the toxic effects of the amphetamines. Thus, small doses produced mainly physical toxic symptoms in Case 1, and mainly psychotic symptoms in Case 2, while in Cases 3 and 4 large doses gave rise to the same type of contrasting pictures. Furthermore, in Case 5 a very large dose resulted in a very mild toxic state, whereas in Case 6 a much smaller dose proved fatal. It is clear, therefore, that in some individuals (Cases 1, 3, and 6) toxic doses of amphetamines produce a primarily physical syndrome very similar to that seen in children, while in others (Cases 2 and 4) the physical symptoms are minimal and instead a true toxic psychosis develops.

The relative frequency of the various physical and mental symptoms is shown in Table VII. This table includes only those cases for which a reasonably complete individual history was available. It excludes 22 of the total number of cases, all of which were instances of solely psychotic reactions. It can be seen that tachycardia was present in 20 of the 32 cases, restlessness and mental excitation in 16, mydriasis and hypertension in 11, anxiety and respiratory disturbances such as hyperpnea and dyspnea in 10, headache in 9, and sweating, weakness, hallucinations and/or delusions, and loss of consciousness or coma in 8. Six cases were fatal.

Thus, when amphetamine intoxication results in a primarily physical syndrome the symptoms are essentially those of sympathetic overstimulation accompanied by such signs of central nervous system stimulation as restlessness and anxiety. On the other hand, when amphetamine intoxication gives rise to a primarily mental syndrome it is characterized by vivid auditory and visual hallucinations and by delusions of persecution usually without disorientation or confusion, as illustrated by Cases 2 and 4 above. Such syndromes accounted for 30 of a total of 54. Judging by the reports, the majority of these cases presented few if any physical symptoms. In this respect Connell (42), discussing the toxic psychoses due to either acute or chronic consumption of amphetamines, concluded that "there are no physical signs diagnostic of amphetamine intoxication." As a rule, the psychotic symptoms disappear without any special treatment in a matter of days following withdrawal of the drug. Since these paranoid psychotic reactions are indistinguishable from those seen in chronic abusers of amphetamines, the whole question of amphetamine psychoses will be discussed fully in chapter IV dealing with the effects of prolonged abuse of the drugs. However, it may well be emphasized that in certain individuals the intake of one or a few doses of amphetamines can and does produce a transitory psychotic episode. Because of this, Connell (42) considers the amphetamines true hallucinogens, as opposed to alcohol which

TABLE VII

SYMPTOMS OF ACUTE AMPHETAMINE INTOXICATION IN ADULTS

Author	Flushing	Pallor, cyanosis, & clammy skin	Sweating	Fever	Dryness of mouth, thirst	Mydriasis	Tachycardia	Palpitation & cardiac discomfort	Raised B.P.	Hemorrhage, vascular accidents	Anorexia, nausea, vomiting	Hyperpnea, dyspnea	Hyperactive reflexes, tremor, ataxia	Twitchings, tetany	Paresthesia, numbness, tingling	Restlessness, mental excitation	Euphoria	Logorrhea	Insomnia	Inebriation	Giddiness	Headache	Weakness, fatigue	Anxiety	Confusion, irrationality	Hallucinations, delusions	Convulsions	Weak pulse, cardiovascular collapse	Loss of consciousness, coma	Death	Duration
Anderson & Scott	×	×					×	×			×	×																×			24 hr.
Davies		×			×	×		×			×					×	×		×		×	×						×			days
Davies									×							×															?
Apfelberg						×		×	×																		×		×		?
Ehrich, et al.							×	×	×															×	×						?
Issekutz						× ×					× ×	×			×	× ×	×	×	× ×		× ×		× ×								10 days
Smith																												×	×	×	2 days
Pous Chazaro																×	×	×	×					×			×				2 days
Pontrelli		×	×		×		×					×				×													×	×	12 hr.
Carratalá & Calzetta			× ×	×							×	×	×	×		×													×		7 days
Gericke		×					×															×	×		×	×				×	12 hr.
Hernandez & Dalmau							× × ×	×	× ×					×	×	×								× ×	×	× ×					3 days / 24 hr.
Curry							×	×												×	×	×	×	× ×	×		×				?
Hart		×					×	×																							24 hr.
Harvey, et al.	×			×			×					×	×													×		×	×	×	3 days
Wallis, et al.							×				×	×	×													×		×	×		24 hr.

TABLE VII (concld.)

Author	Flushing	Pallor, cyanosis, & clammy skin	Sweating	Fever	Dryness of mouth, thirst	Mydriasis	Tachycardia	Palpitation & cardiac discomfort	Raised B.P.	Hemorrhage, vascular accidents	Anorexia, nausea, vomiting	Hyperpnea, dyspnea	Hyperactive reflexes, tremor, ataxia	Twitchings, tetany	Paresthesia, numbness, tingling	Restlessness, mental excitation	Euphoria	Logorrhea	Insomnia	Inebriation	Giddiness	Headache	Weakness, fatigue	Anxiety	Confusion, irrationality	Hallucinations, delusions	Convulsions	Weak pulse, cardiovascular collapse	Loss of consciousness, coma	Death	Duration
Temkin		×					×	×												×	×	×	×	×							24 hr.
Ruiz Ogara		×			×	×	×	×	×	×						×								×		×			×		2 days
Fedeli & Lumia			×													×						×					×				8 days
Poteliakhoff & Roughton									× ×				×		×		×					× ×									5 wk. / 24 hr.
Pathy		×				×	×			×	×	×				×				×	×		×		×						24 hr.
Greenwood & Peachy	×		×		×	× × ×	× × ×	×	× × ×		×	×	×	×		× ×							×	× ×	×	×					3 days / 24 hr. / 3 days
Vill		×		×			×									×															days
Ayache				×								×				×		×				×		×		×					24 hr.
Bernheim & Cox				×			×					×																×	×	×	5 hr.
Jordan & Hampson				×		×	×															×						×	×	×	4 hr.
Tonks and Livingston	×		×				×						×									×	×						×		5 days
TOTALS FOR 32 CASES	4	8	8	6	4	11	20	9	11	2	7	10	5	3	3	16	5	3	5	3	6	9	8	10	7	8	4	6	8	6	

produces hallucinoses only after a long period of excessive drinking.

According to Connell (42) the minimum dose capable of producing psychotic symptoms is 50 mg, although he adds: "In theory, a person could be so sensitive to the drug that psychotic symptoms occur with low doses, but this has not been reported, the lowest dose being stated as 50 mg." Although in most of the cases here reviewed the doses were larger than 50 mg, in at least two instances they were smaller. Thus, Carratala and Calzetta (37) reported a psychotic reaction in a woman produced by 30 mg of methamphetamine hydrochloride, and in 1954 Ruiz Ogara (156) reported a similar episode following the intravenous administration of 10 mg of amphetamine. It will also be recalled that Lancer (113) reported visual hallucinations in a 5-year-old child who had taken 15 mg of d-amphetamine over a period of 3 days. Thus, marked sensitivity to the toxic effects of amphetamines does exist and this also applies to the physical effects, as illustrated by Temkin's case described above. The opposite, of course, is equally true: certain individuals, as in Case 5 above, can take large doses of amphetamines without marked effects, either physical or mental.

Both the intensity and the quality of the toxic symptoms depend therefore not only on the dose of amphetamine taken but also on the mental and physical characteristics of the individual. This raises the interesting question of which factors in the make-up of an individual determine these various patterns of response. Research along this line does not appear to have been carried out to date. In general, however, as shown in Table VI, the doses capable of producing a toxic state were many times the usual therapeutic dose.

Six of the 54 cases listed in Table VI were fatal (169, 143, 70, 90, 24, and 104). In one of these cases (90) death apparently resulted from acute hepatic necrosis. Since amphetamines are not generally thought to be hepatotoxic, and since this patient was an alcoholic with extensive fatty infiltration of the liver, it is difficult to know what role amphetamine played in his death. Amphetamine appears to be more clearly implicated in the remaining 5 cases. Two of these deaths were attributable to hyperpyrexia (21 and 104), 2 of the patients died of intracranial complications (143 and 70), and in the fifth case (169) there was sudden cardiovascular collapse unexplained by any anatomical finding at autopsy and therefore conceivably due to ventricular fibrillation. These cases are too few and varied to permit any generalization. However, acute toxicity studies in animals (56 and 57) indicate that death results from excessive sympathomimetic activity, and the findings in at least 5 of these 6 cases are compatible with such an explanation.

Milder forms of amphetamine toxicity are also produced by therapeutic doses of these drugs in many individuals, but are usually considered as side effects and consist of similar but much less severe signs of stimulation of the sympathetic and central nervous systems. Side effect, is, of course, a very ambiguous term, meaning essentially an undesirable effect produced by what is normally a therapeutic dose for a specific purpose. Thus, insomnia may be considered a side effect when decrease in appetite is the main objective, or anorexia when a decrease in the need for sleep is the aim. An extensive and detailed description of these side effects has been provided recently by Welsh (191), but one of the best evaluations is still the early study by Jacobsen, *et al.* (18, 102, and 103), involving several hundred normal healthy members of the general population engaged in their usual daily activities.

Naturally, experiments in man with frankly toxic doses of the amphetamines are extremely rare. In 1938, however, Waud (189) reported on a series of 8 experiments carried out at 6- to 10-day intervals on a normal man weighing 213 pounds. Each experiment consisted of the continuous inhalation of the contents of 2 amphetamine inhalers for 4 to 6 hours and the observation and recording of the effects produced. The amphetamine base content of the two inhalers was 650 mg and the estimated amount absorbed was 400–500 mg. This was approximately 1000 times the usual therapeutic dose by inhalation. The most prominent symptoms noted were dilatation of the pupils lasting for 6–12 hours and sluggish reaction to light and accommodation; extreme dryness of the mouth and pharynx for 24 hours; extreme soreness of the throat on three occasions; moderate dyspnea on exertion for 72 hours; many extrasystoles for 4–5 days and paroxysmal tachycardia on two occasions at the end of inhalation; unstable heart rhythm and presence of sinus arrhythmia; marked tachycardia on exertion and moderate tachycardia at rest for 2 days; hypertension for 24 hours after inhalation, extreme loss of appetite for 48 to 60 hours leading to a loss of 10 to 14 pounds (regained in one week); extreme flatulence for 60 hours and marked abdominal distension for 48 hours; constipation for 4–5 days; marked coldness and blanching of extremities with marked flushing of the face and neck for 24 to 48 hours; marked tingling of the skin during and after the experiment; increased mental activity with decrease in mental efficiency during inhalation; decrease in memory for 2 to 3 days; marked insomnia for 48 to 72 hours; moderate euphoria during inhalation, followed by secondary mental depression and fatigue for several days; coarse tremor of the hands and moderately increased reflexes for 24 hours.

It is evident from this description that Waud's subject reacted to large doses of amphetamine base with primarily physical symptoms of the type listed in Table VII, and of only moderate degree. Waud concluded, among other things, that the margin of safety of the drug is great in normal persons. This conclusion is obviously unwarranted since it was based on observations on a single subject. The apparent lack of correlation between dose and intensity of reaction, evident in the 54 cases reviewed here, would suggest rather that there is a wide range of individual variation in sensitivity to the toxic effects of the amphetamines. However, since most of those subjects were not normal in the strict sense of the term, the range of sensitivity shown by them may not be valid for a normal population.

In addition to uncomplicated acute amphetamine intoxication there is also the risk of poisoning by the combined use of monoamine oxidase inhibitors and pressor amines such as the amphetamines, as illustrated by the reports of Tonks and Livingston (177) and Roecker and Lane (152). It is apparent that the monoamine oxidase inhibitors potentiate the action of the pressor amines, so that toxic symptoms appear with much smaller doses. This matter is currently receiving a good deal of attention in the medical literature (122, 50, 138, 33, and 58).

With respect to the frequency with which acute amphetamine intoxication occurs in adults, all that can be concluded with certainty from this review is that a minimum of 54 cases has been reported since 1939. Examination of Table VI strongly suggests, however, that this figure bears little if any relation to the true incidence. It is rather remarkable, for example, that 26 out of a total of 54 cases were reported in Great Britain; that 19 of these 26 reports appeared between 1956 and 1958; and that 13 of the latter were observed by a single author over a 3-year period (42). Table VI also shows that all of the cases from the United States were published prior to 1954. These figures suggest either a very uneven incidence of intoxications at different periods in different countries, or, what is more probable, a lack of consistency between the frequency of these cases and their appearance in the medical literature. Two factors may contribute to this erratic reporting. In the first place cases of acute amphetamine poisoning presenting with primarily physical symptoms and treated in general hospitals are considered routine. Jordan and Hampson (104), for example, were prompted to report a fatal case in 1960 because of an editorial in the *British Medical Journal* (5) dealing with the problem of hyperpyrexia in cases of amphetamine intoxication. It was clearly implied that the case would not have been published otherwise. Secondly, a substantial number of these cases, as Table VI shows, displayed an acute psychotic reaction hardly distinguishable from paranoid schizophrenia. These cases are generally admitted to psychiatric hospitals and often misdiagnosed (42) unless a proper history is available or, as rarely happens, chemical determination of amphetamines in the urine is performed.

Inquiries at one large teaching hospital in the city of Toronto revealed only one case diagnosed as amphetamine poisoning in the period 1953–63. But the lack of published reports from this country should not lead one to the conclusion that the problem does not exist.

Summary

Fifty-four cases of acute and subacute amphetamine intoxication were found in the literature. Six cases were fatal. In five instances the drugs were taken on medical prescription; in the remainder they were self-administered for various purposes, including attempted suicide. The amounts taken ranged from 5 to 630 mg of *d*-amphetamine, but in most cases they were many times the therapeutic dose. This indicates both wide individual variability in response and a relatively wide margin of safety.

In more than half of the cases the toxic picture consisted primarily of a transitory psychotic reaction, with auditory and visual hallucinations and delusions of persecution, and relatively minor physical symptoms. In the remainder, the picture was one of overstimulation of the central and sympathetic nervous systems. The most frequent symptoms were tachycardia, restlessness and mental excitation, mydriasis, hypertension, anxiety, respiratory disturbances, and headache. Mono-amine oxidase inhibitors potentiate the action of amphetamines so that toxic symptoms appear with much smaller doses.

The erratic distribution of case reports with respect to time and country, together with the difficulty in establishing the diagnosis in cases with predominantly psychotic symptoms, suggest that the incidence of amphetamine poisoning may be far greater than the number of published reports would indicate.

III. Toxic Effects due to Chronic
Consumption of Amphetamines

CERTAIN CONDITIONS, such as narcolepsy or obesity, are sometimes treated with prolonged daily use of amphetamines. In these instances the drugs should be taken under medical supervision so that dosage, length of medication, and other factors are under the control of the physician who can observe the appearance of toxic symptoms and alter the treatment accordingly. But some of the actions of these drugs on the central nervous system, such as their analeptic and euphoriant effects, made them from the start very widely sought for non-medical purposes by the general public. This led on the one hand to abuse of the amphetamines by some individuals, and on the other to more or less stringent legislation in various countries designed to curtail the abuse.

The literature concerning the extent of abuse of these drugs, as well as on its consequences, is extremely controversial, poorly documented, and in many instances markedly biased, perhaps because the amphetamines induce some highly desirable beneficial effects on man, and because the toxic or undesirable effects are not as dramatic or as easily defined as those of such other psychotropic drugs as the narcotics.

The question of whether or not the amphetamines are addictive drugs has received a great deal of attention and much has been written on both sides of the issue. The discussion of this problem has developed into an almost futile semantic exercise, in the meantime obscuring the fact that the chronic use of a drug may have highly undesirable consequences without necessarily producing addiction according to one or another definition of the term. It has already been shown that even a single therapeutic dose of amphetamine can cause a psychotic episode in certain individuals. In this chapter it will be shown that prolonged abuse has led to psychotic reactions of a schizophrenic type in many individuals, regardless of whether or not they could properly be called addicts. Thus, although the question of the addictive properties of these drugs is an important one, it should not be allowed to obscure the other possible undesirable consequences of their chronic abuse. Habitual use of a psychotropic drug for non-medical reasons is in itself a sign of abnormal behavior, but that problem is beyond the scope of this review, since it deals with the causes rather than the consequences of taking certain drugs.

The question of addiction *per se* will be dealt with in chapter v.

In this and the following chapters, the literature concerning the ill effects of prolonged use of amphetamines will be reviewed as exhaustively as possible. Ideally such a review should answer at least three major questions. (1) What ill effects, if any, does the chronic use of amphetamines produce? (2) What is the incidence of chronic misuse? (3) In what proportion of all cases are there undesirable effects? The literature provides a reasonably satisfactory answer to the first question since it refers essentially to a qualitative problem. Unfortunately, the second and third questions cannot be answered from the data available in the medical literature, although some educated guesses can be made. It will be apparent from this review that in order to find out what the frequency of chronic amphetamine consumption is in any given community, and what consequences this has for the individual and the community, a specific and proper survey should be carried out.

CHRONIC CONSUMPTION OF AMPHETAMINES WITHOUT ILL EFFECTS

It is next to impossible to judge from the literature how many people take amphetamines habitually without suffering any ill effects, since obviously such people do not usually report their experience. However, as the following cases show, these drugs can be taken for long periods of time without producing either any appreciable toxic effects, or, in the opinion of some authors, addiction.

In 1938 Lesses and Myerson (117) claimed that after more than two years of extensive clinical experience with amphetamines they had not seen a single case of addiction "in the sense that a person, otherwise well, now feels it necessary to take the drug habitually and in ascending doses to produce a desired effect." After two more years of experience with the drugs Myerson (131) still held the same view. Guttmann (80), summarizing his experience with amphetamines in psychiatric practice, reported only one case referred with a diagnosis of addiction, and he did not consider it to be so in the strict sense of the term.

In 1940 Bloomberg (28) reported the results of a clinical and laboratory investigation on 3 narcoleptics. Two of them had been taking 70 mg of amphetamine sulfate daily for 2 years and 8 months and the other, a 62-year-old man, had been taking the same dose for 1 year and 8 months. These patients were thoroughly studied in the hospital for 3 days and no significant abnormality was found. None of them had had to increase the dose and one had been able to lower it. Furthermore, they were all able to stop taking the drug during the period of observation without showing any signs of craving. Bloomberg adds that having treated "a great number of alcoholic patients" with amphetamine, he had seen no important untoward side effects, development of tolerance, or signs of habituation or addiction. He also cited the case of a patient who took 150 mg of the drug by mistake over a period of 14 hours and suffered nothing worse than a sleepless night and irritability for about 36 hours.

An interesting case is that reported by Bakst (19). A 36-year-old seaman had been taking 15–30 mg of amphetamine sulfate daily for 9 years because of an original diagnosis of narcolepsy. When the patient was re-examined and kept under observation for 15 days without receiving amphetamine, the diagnosis of narcolepsy could not be supported. The author concluded: "No remarkable effects of the long continued usage of the drug could be demonstrated, nor were any perceptible changes noted when the drug was discontinued." A few years later Finch (62) claimed to have used d-amphetamine in the treatment of over 400 patients, including a large group of obese cases, and never to have found anyone who craved the drug or who refused to discontinue it.

More recently Grahn (75), reporting on his experience with amphetamines in private practice, provided the following information: of 32 patients who had received amphetamines for as long as 16 years, 15 had a definite medical indication for the drug but took it only when they could not do without it. The others showed some signs of habituation but were able to give up the drug without much difficulty. One man with postencephalitic parkinsonism, who had been treated with amphetamines for 16 years, took 60 mg of d-amphetamine daily during work days, but did not take any during weekends, when he slept for most of the 48 hours. Grahn claims to have seen only one case that could properly be considered addiction to amphetamines. Leake (116) gives further references dealing with the relative lack of toxicity of the amphetamines in the course of the chronic treatment of various conditions.

These examples show that the amphetamines can be taken in considerable doses and for prolonged periods by some individuals without any marked physical or mental toxic effects. They also show that chronic intake does not necessarily lead to the development of habituation or addiction. However, a significant number of reports indicate that in certain individuals prolonged consumption of amphetamines does give rise to toxic effects and/or a strong dependency on these drugs. Although in many instances these two problems overlap, they will be discussed separately.

CHRONIC CONSUMPTION OF AMPHETAMINES WITH TOXIC EFFECTS

Regardless of the purpose or reason for which amphetamines may be consumed chronically, various sorts of toxic effects have been described, of which the most severe and dramatic is the development of a schizophrenia-like psychosis. By far the most widespread and serious problem due to the chronic abuse of the amphetamines developed in Japan after the end of the second world war (see chapter v). A search of the literature outside Japan has revealed a total of 242 case reports dealing with the toxic effects of prolonged consumption of amphetamines. Of these cases, 201 or 83 per cent suffered one or more psychotic episodes of a schizophrenic type which were clearly related to the consumption of amphetamines. This problem will be considered separately in the next chapter. In the remaining 41 cases, the toxic symptoms ranged from dermatitis to severe anxiety states.

Thus, Goldsmith (74) described a case of skin eruption in a narcoleptic woman being treated with amphetamine. Kauvar, *et al.* (107), reported the case of a woman who developed a pruritic lichenified eruption of the skin a few days after being put on a regimen for weight control that included 10 mg of amphetamine sulfate daily. Every time that the drug was discontinued the dermatitis disappeared. Other cases of dermatitis associated with prolonged consumption of amphetamines have been reported by Howard (98), McCormick (127), and Welsh (191).

In 1950 Mitchell and Denton (128) reported a fatal case of panhemocytopenia in a 21-year-old nurse, which was attributed by the authors to the consumption of massive doses of *d*-amphetamine sulfate. No other case of this nature appears to have been reported. Other unique cases of amphetamine toxicity are those reported by Atkinson (15) and by Julien and Vincendeau (105). In the first, a picture of simulated thyrotoxicosis was attributed to the combined prolonged intake of *d*-amphetamine sulfate and thyroid extract, and in the second, a case of heterochromia of Fuchs was thought to be related to the abuse of amphetamine.

Various toxic states including the characteristic symptoms of overdosage of amphetamines such as sympathetic overstimulation, anorexia, insomnia, irritability, and hyperactivity have been reported by Gayral and Combes (69), Knapp (110), Baruk and Joubert (20), Corni (44), Zondek (202), and Askevold (14). In all these cases amphetamines had been consumed for periods ranging from 2 to 15 years, in maximum daily doses of from 50 to 450 mg.

The largest series in this group is that reported by McConnell and McIlwaine (126) and McConnell (125) from Northern Ireland. These authors state that over a period of 28 months they saw 25 cases of toxic states associated with the abuse of amphetamines. Twenty of the patients had become dependent on these drugs and, when seen, they were all agitated and depressed despite increased dosage. Two of the other 5 patients, one being treated for dysmenorrhea and another for depression, developed anxiety, tension, and restlessness while receiving the drug. Another patient, who had amphetamine prescribed because of memory loss and poor concentration, became tense and anxious and his original complaints became worse. A fourth patient who received amphetamines for apathy and tiredness suddenly developed severe headache and copious vomiting. In all cases the symptoms disappeared rapidly on withdrawal of the drug.

The toxic effects noted above may be divided into three categories. One consists of a small group of evidently allergic reactions or idiosyncrasies (e.g., blood dyscrasias, dermatitis) such as are seen with a very wide variety of drugs and are therefore of no specific interest with respect to the amphetamines. The second group consists of an even smaller number of most unusual disturbances, such as the heterochromia of Fuchs, which were only suspected of being the results of amphetamine ingestion. Since a causal relation was not proven, these cases are of only minor interest. The third and largest group showed symptoms such as anxiety, restlessness, anorexia, and insomnia which are the typical effects of amphetamine and are virtually the same as the acute toxic effects noted previously. The psychic and emotional disturbances in these patients may well represent the initial stages of development of amphetamine psychosis.

SUMMARY

Many reports indicate that amphetamines may be used therapeutically for long periods of time without modification of dosage and without untoward effects. However, there are also numerous reports of chronic use resulting in various ill effects. The most important of these is a toxic psychosis. The remaining cases presented a heterogeneous collection of physical and mental toxic symptoms, most of which represented exaggerations of the characteristic effects of the drug.

IV. Amphetamine Psychosis

A PSYCHOTIC REACTION closely resembling paranoid schizophrenia appears to be the most frequent and serious toxic manifestation associated with the chronic consumption of amphetamines. This conclusion is borne out by the literature in which 201 of 242 cases of chronic toxicity suffered from psychotic illness.

Young and Scoville (200), as early as 1938 in a paper entitled "Paranoid Psychosis in Narcolepsy and the Possible Danger of Benzedrine Treatment," were the first to call attention to the possible link between chronic consumption of amphetamine and psychotic illness. Three years later Staehelin (170) reported a case of methamphetamine psychosis in Switzerland and noted its similarity to the better known cocaine psychoses. During the same year Greving (78) described 2 cases of the same type in Germany and remarked that the toxic mental symptoms associated with prolonged abuse of methamphetamine were suggestive of mescaline action. In 1942 Daube (52) presented a series of 4 patients in whom prolonged methamphetamine abuse led to the following psychotic symptoms: illusions and hallucinations of all sensory modalities, loosely systematized ideas of reference and of influence, and marked anxiety. His patients retained normal orientation and consciousness, however.

Despite these early reports, a relatively small number of cases had appeared in the literature until 1958 when Connell published his *Amphetamine Psychosis* (42). He states that a search of the English and French literature revealed authenticated reports of 36 cases up to 1956, including those associated with acute amphetamine intoxication. The present search of the literature, which includes as many cases as could be found, has revealed 71 cases up to the time Connell's book appeared. Of these, 15 were instances of psychotic reactions associated with acute amphetamine intoxication and have already been described. In view of the widespread use of the amphetamines and of the number of years they have been available, these figures would suggest that amphetamine psychosis is a rare condition.

Struck by the close resemblance between the mental symptoms in amphetamine psychosis and those seen in paranoid schizophrenia, Connell thought that perhaps "errors of diagnosis might often occur with patients taking amphetamine-like drugs, particularly since drug addicts frequently deny addiction or falsify the amounts taken, even after voluntarily seeking advice" (p. 11). An investigation covering a three-year period (1953–56) and including patients seen in five London hospitals led to the discovery of 42 cases of amphetamine psychosis. Although another 14 cases came to the author's attention they were not included in the study for practical reasons. Connell remarks: "It was not expected to find many patients, since the condition, as judged by the relevant literature, appeared to be rare in this country. It was a surprise, therefore, to discover how prevalent is the habit of taking amphetamine, and how common a resulting psychotic illness."

The literature on amphetamine psychosis published since 1958 has amply confirmed Connell's finding that the incidence of this syndrome is far greater than was hitherto suspected. Thus, during the five-year period from 1958 to June, 1963, 118 cases have been reported (excluding the 42 cases reported by Connell) as opposed to 71 in the 20 years following Young and Scoville's first report. Even more significant is the fact that the recent literature includes many examples of large series seen by one author or by a group of authors. The following are examples: Askevold (14), 1959, 7 cases from Norway; Beamish and Kiloh (21), 1960, 6 cases from England; Bell and Trethowan (22 and 23), 1961, 14 cases from Australia; Hampton (85), 1961, 31 cases from the United States; Rickman, et al. (150), 1961, 18 cases from the United States; and Grantham, et al. (76), 1962, 4 cases from Canada. These clusters of cases seen by individual groups of investigators in different parts of the world during the last few years indicate either that the incidence of amphetamine psychosis is increasing, or that the condition has been almost unrecognized until recently.

Since Connell's study of amphetamine psychosis is the most thorough and comprehensive, his findings will be summarized and the other cases reported in the literature assessed in terms of his conclusions.

DESCRIPTION BY CONNELL

The clinical material consisted of 42 cases which Connell classified into 3 groups:

1. Those who took single doses of the drug only (8 cases).
2. Those who had also been taking alcohol at the time of the development of the psychosis (4 cases).
3. Those who had been taking regular doses of the drug for more than a month (30 cases).

Although useful from certain points of view, such as addiction, this classification appears to be of little significance from the standpoint of the psychoses described, and the discussion that follows refers, therefore, to the whole group unless otherwise specified.

Most of the patients were young adults with a tendency to poor marital history and a rather high incidence of previous mental illness. There was frequently a family history of mental illness. About two-thirds of the patients had presented neurotic traits in childhood, antisocial activities, and poor work records. Connell considers that "this is only to be expected, since persons with abnormal personalities are much more likely to become drug addicts than are normal people." However, since the group included some patients with apparently normal personalities and backgrounds, and since the majority were friendly and outgoing rather than introverted and suspicious, Connell rejects the view of some authors (200, 130, 135, and 39) that amphetamine psychosis is merely an exaggeration of latent paranoid traits.

Most of the patients had begun taking the drugs to combat fatigue, lack of energy, or depression, but a few had used them because of obesity. Almost a quarter of the patients developed psychoses after a single dose or a short period of intake, but the remainder had been using the drugs for long periods of time. The daily doses varied widely, ranging from 20 mg of d-amphetamine sulfate to 985 mg of amphetamine base (equivalent to 1687 mg of amphetamine sulfate), the most common dose being 325 mg of the base (that is, the contents of one inhaler). In some cases prolonged heavy use without symptoms was followed by a psychosis when the dose was only slightly increased. All of the amphetamines were represented, and in most cases the drug was taken orally. The principal effects noted by the chronic drug users were the characteristic ones, including increased energy, cheerfulness, talkativeness, anorexia, thirst, dry mouth, insomnia, and depression on withdrawal. Contrary to usual reports, libido was not consistently affected. The only physical signs seen on admission were the characteristic sympathomimetic consequences of the drug. Connell does not consider these signs to be of diagnostic significance, because they could also have resulted from extreme anxiety.

Most patients were referred because of severe disturbances of behavior, including violence, suicidal attempts, and requests for police protection. There was a striking similarity among all the patients with respect to the clinical picture with a high frequency of persecutory ideas. Most were initially diagnosed as paranoid schizophrenics even in instances where the patient was known to have taken amphetamines. Ideas of reference and hallucinations of all sensory modalities were frequent. The absence of disorientation was an important finding because, as Connell points out, it is normally considered characteristic of a toxic state.

After withdrawal of the drug the symptoms cleared rapidly, usually in a week or less. The exact duration was obscured in some patients because they continued to take smuggled drugs while in hospital. Connell therefore recommends the use of chemical tests for amphetamine in the urine in cases where the symptoms do not subside. Depression and sleepiness were the only common withdrawal symptoms. Although no systematic follow-up was attempted, available information and numerous re-admissions suggested a high rate of relapse.

The differential diagnosis of amphetamine psychosis in Connell's opinion should be based mainly on the relation between the clinical picture and the presence of amphetamine in the urine, since there are no specific diagnostic signs or symptoms. Otherwise the psychosis could be, and often is, diagnosed as paranoid schizophrenia, or occasionally as alcoholic or bromide hallucinosis.

Connell ends by advising caution in the prescription of amphetamine and allied drugs, especially for depression and fatigue, since there is no reliable means for recognizing subjects who are liable to become addicted.

CLINICAL CHARACTERISTICS OF AMPHETAMINE PSYCHOSIS

Table VIII lists some pertinent data concerning the reported cases of psychosis associated with chronic consumption of amphetamines. The table is based on all the cases found during the course of this review, including those reported by Connell.

Unfortunately a number of recent papers have dealt with group reports rather than with individual case histories. Even when individual case histories are given they are by no means consistent with one another, since they were written by many authors with different backgrounds, points of view, and interests. Therefore it is impossible to give exact and complete figures for the frequency of various features of the illness. Figures are given in the following text on the basis of whatever information was available; to avoid unnecessary repetition, the total number of cases referred to means all cases listed in Table VIII for which adequate information was available.

Mental Condition During Psychotic Episode

Of the 201 cases of psychotic reactions associated with chronic consumption of amphetamines, 29 were described by Connell and have already been discussed. Of the remaining 172 cases, 78 have been described recently in group reports rather than individually and therefore only general information was available. However, a more detailed study of the 94 cases for which individual case histories were reported has essentially confirmed Connell's findings. Eighty-seven of these cases presented with a paranoid and hallucinatory picture. Their major mental symptoms are listed in

41

TABLE VIII

REPORTED CASES OF PSYCHOSIS ASSOCIATED WITH CHRONIC USE OF AMPHETAMINES

Author	Reference	Sex	Age	Drug*	Maximum daily dose	Duration of use	Other drugs taken to excess
Young & Scoville (1938) U.S.A.	200	M	34	dl-A SO₄	60 mg	months	
		M	25	dl-A SO₄	?	6 wk.	
Greving (1941) Germany	78	M	27	meth-A HCl	215 mg	2.5 yr.	
		M	30	meth-A HCl	270 mg	2.5 yr.	
Staehelin (1941) Switzerland	170	M	28	meth-A HCl	150 mg	months	alcohol
Daube (1942) Germany	52	F	24	meth-A HCl	75 mg	1 yr.	analgesics; caffeine
		M	35	meth-A HCl	60 mg	3 yr.	morphine; barbiturates
		M	37	meth-A HCl	4 ampoules (parenteral)	6 mo.	morphine; cocaine
		M	56	meth-A HCl	180 mg (oral, parenteral, sniffing)	2 yr.	morphine; cocaine
Hartmann (1942) Switzerland	89	M	35	meth-A HCl	75 mg	3 yr.	morphine
Norman & Shea (1945) U.S.A.	134	M	49	dl-A SO₄	250 mg	6 yr.	alcohol
Shorvon (1945) U.K.	165	M	35	dl-A SO₄	150 mg	5 yr.	
Hagenau & Aubrun (1947) France	81	F	52	dl-A SO₄	700 mg	5 yr.	
Harder (1947) Germany	87	M	33	dl-A SO₄; meth-A HCl	600 mg	4 yr.	coffee
		M	35	meth-A HCl	270 mg	3 yr.	alcohol, heroin
Hernandez & Dalmau (1948) Puerto Rico	93	M	33	dl-A	250 mg	?	alcohol
Schneck (1948) U.S.A.	159	M	26	dl-A	375 mg	?	
Brown (1949) U.S.A.	32	M	?	dl-A	1250 mg	?	alcohol
		M	?	dl-A	?	?	marihuana
		M	38	dl-A	750 mg	12 yr.	alcohol
Freyhan (1949) U.S.A.	67	M	40	dl-A	250 mg	?	alcohol

TABLE VIII (cont.)

Author	Reference	Sex	Age	Drug*	Maximum daily dose	Duration of use	Other drugs taken to excess
Peterson & Somerville (1949) Australia	142	M	29	dl-A SO₄	375 mg	6 yr.	alcohol; cocaine; heroin
Heuyer & Lebovici (1950) France	95	M	33	d-A tartrate	800 mg (I.V.)	6 mo.	morphine
		M	45	d-A tartrate	?	?	morphine; cocaine; barbiturates
O'Flanagan & Taylor (1950) U.K.	135	M	38	dl-A; dl-A SO₄	650 mg	6 yr.	
Nandelstadh (1951) ?	132	M	27	dl-A	?	2 yr.	
		M	45	meth-A	?	2 yr.	
		M	30	dl-A	?	6.5 yr.	alcohol; sedatives
Knapp (1952) U.S.A.	110	F	22	dl-A SO₄	90 mg	6 mo.	
Alliez (1953) France	3	F	21	dl-A SO₄	200 mg (I.M.)	2 yr.	
Baruk & Joubert (1953) France	20	M	45	dl-A SO₄; d-A tartrate	120 mg (I.V.)	?	morphine
Pottier, et al. (1953) France	145	M	34	dl-A SO₄; d-A tartrate	200 mg	2 yr.	
Bonhoff & Lewrenz (1954) Germany	29	M	29	meth-A HCl	? (parenteral)	years	Dolantin
		M	28	meth-A HCl	90 mg	4 yr.	Isophen; caffeine
		M	48	meth-A HCl	?	8 yr.	sedatives; coffee; Cardiazol; Dicodid
Carr (1954) U.K.	36	M	41	meth-A	1250 mg	?	
Chapman (1954) U.S.A.	39	M	32	dl-A SO₄	30 mg	4 yr.	
		M	39	dl-A SO₄	90 mg	4 mo.	alcohol
Delay, et al. (1954) France	54	F	29	dl-A SO₄	750 mg	5 yr.	
		M	29	d-A tartrate	416 mg	?	alcohol
		F	21	d-A tartrate	?	6 yr.	

TABLE VIII (cont.)

Author	Reference	Sex	Age	Drug*	Maximum daily dose	Duration of use	Other drugs taken to excess
Herman & Nagler (1954) U.S.A.	92	F	23	dl-A	500 mg	1 yr.	alcohol; marihuana; morphine; cocaine
		M	31	dl-A	250 mg	1 mo.	
		M	37	dl-A	250 mg	?	alcohol; morphine; heroin
		M	37	dl-A	250 mg	1 mo.	alcohol
Schinko & Solms (1954) Austria	158	F	30	meth-A tartrate	150 mg	2.5 yr.	
Martimor, et al. (1955) France	120	M	38	d-A tartrate	500 mg (I.V.)	months	
Simpson (1957) U.S.A.	168	F	33	meth-A HCl; thyroid, atropine, alloin & phenobarbital	30 mg	4 yr.	
Tolentino & D'Avossa (1957) Italy	176	F	23	meth-A HCl	30 mg	4 yr.	
		M	36	dl-A SO4; meth-A HCl	60 tablets	16 yr.	
		M	39	d-A SO4	20 tablets	7 yr.	morphine
		M	31	d-A SO4	3 vials	10 yr.	
		M	27	d-A SO4	?	3 mo.	
		M	48	meth-A HCl	?	2 yr. +	morphine
		M	48	dl-A SO4	60 tablets	7 yr.	
Wallis (1957) U.K.	185	M	20	dl-A	650 mg	?	alcohol
Connell (1958) U.K.	42	F	42	d-A SO4	250 mg	more than 1 month	
		M	41	d-A SO4	50 mg	more than 1 month	
		M	45	dl-A SO4	?	more than 1 month	
		M	39	d-A	325 mg	more than 1 month	
		M	22	d-A SO4	?	more than 1 month	
		M	45	d-A SO4	150 mg	more than 1 month	
		M	21	dl-A	325 mg	more than 1 month	
		M	49	dl-A	650 mg	more than 1 month	
		F	29	d-A SO4	30 mg	more than 1 month	
		F	22	d-A SO4	100 mg	more than 1 month	
		F	28	d-A SO4	60 mg	more than 1 month	
		F	48	d-A SO4	?	more than 1 month	

TABLE VIII (cont.)

Author	Reference	Sex	Age	Drug*	Maximum daily dose	Duration of use	Other drugs taken to excess
		M	31	dl-A SO₄	250 mg	more than 1 month	
		F	35	dl-A SO₄	20 mg ?	more than 1 month	
		M	21	dl-A	250 mg	more than 1 month	
		M	28	dl-A	325 mg	more than 1 month	
		M	37	meth-A	70 mg	more than 1 month	
		M	30	dl-A	325 mg	more than 1 month	
		F	22	dl-A	325 mg	more than 1 month	
		F	32	dl-A	325 mg	more than 1 month	
		M	35	dl-A SO₄	60 mg	more than 1 month	
		M	34	d-A SO₄	50 mg	more than 1 month	
		M	25	d-A SO₄	20 mg	more than 1 month	
		F	45	dl-A SO₄	200 mg	more than 1 month	
		M	37	d-A SO₄	150 mg	more than 1 month	
		F	41	d-A SO₄	150 mg	more than 1 month	
		F	23	d-A SO₄	75 mg	more than 1 month	
		M	32	dl-A	975 mg	more than 1 month	
		F	24	dl-A	975 mg	more than 1 month	
Grahn (1958) U.S.A.	75	F	?	dl-A SO₄; d-A SO₄	100 mg	?	
Tolentino (1958) Italy	175	M	44	meth-A HCl; dl-A SO₄	30 tablets	12 yr.	Allypropymal
		M	45	dl-A SO₄	25 tablets	months	alcohol
Askevold (1959) Norway	14	M	37	amphetamine	500 mg	5 yr.	alcohol
		M	36	amphetamine	100 mg	months	barbiturates
		M	53	amphetamine	200 mg	years	alcohol; morphine, barbiturates
		M	39	amphetamine	?	years	
		M	51	amphetamine	100 mg	2 yr.	
		M	28	amphetamine	50 mg	years	barbiturates
		M	49	amphetamine	150 mg	4 yr.	barbiturates
Fischer (1959) Australia	63	M	27	dl-A SO₄	600 mg	weeks	phenmetrazine
Abely, et al. (1960) France	1	F	29	d-A tartrate	?	years	phenmetrazine
		F	19	d-A tartrate	?	2 yr.	

TABLE VIII (cont.)

Author	Reference	Sex	Age	Drug*	Maximum daily dose	Duration of use	Other drugs taken to excess
Beamish & Kiloh (1900) U.K.	21	M	37	dl-A SO₄; d-A SO₄	?	17 yr.	Personnia; Chlorodyne; phenmetrazine
		M	39	meth-A HCl	100 mg	5 yr.	mist.pot.brom. et chloral; barbiturates; phen-metrazine
		F	32	d-A SO₄	?	5 yr.	pethidine; phen-metrazine; morphine; promethazine
		M	35	d-A SO₄	300 mg	2 yr.	barbiturates
		M	30	d-A SO₄	?	3 yr.	
		M	36	d-A SO₄; pentobarbital	125 mg 750 mg	4 yr. +	
Ferrero (1960) Argentina	61	F	27	dl-A SO₄	20 tablets	?	
Marley (1960) U.K.	119	M	40	meth-A HCl	?	1 yr.	alcohol; barbiturates, carbromal; Oblivon
		M	39	dl-A SO₄	65 mg	2 mo.	barbiturates
		M	55	d-A SO₄	30 mg	8 mo.	
		F	25	d-A SO₄	150 mg	2 yr.	barbiturates; codeine; morphine
		M	48	d-A SO₄	25 mg	3 mo.	alcohol
		M	35	dl-A SO₄	250 mg	3 mo.	barbiturates; morphine pethidine
Bell & Trethowan (1961) Australia	22	M	49	dl-A SO₄; d-A SO₄; meth-A HCl	1000 mg	6 yr.	alcohol
		F	22	dl-A SO₄; d-A SO₄; meth-A HCl	400 mg	7 yr.	alcohol; phenmetrazine; caffeine, morphine
		M	32	dl-A SO₄; d-A SO₄	175 mg	5 yr.	barbiturates
		M	36	dl-A SO₄; d-A SO₄	200 mg	6 yr.	alcohol; bromides
		M	29	dl-A SO₄; d-A SO₄	150 mg	10 yr.	alcohol
		F	26	d-A SO₄; meth-A HCl	150 mg	4 yr.	
		F	38	d-A SO₄; dl-A SO₄	150 mg	10 yr.	bromides; aspirin-caffeine

TABLE VIII (concld.)

Author	Reference	Sex	Age	Drug*	Maximum daily dose	Duration of use	Other drugs taken to excess
Hampton (1961) U.S.A.	85	F	32	d-A SO₄	30 mg ?	3 yr.	barbiturates
		F	36	dl-A SO₄	50 mg	4 wk.	
		F	32	d-A SO₄	350 mg	6 yr.	phenmetrazine
		M	30	d-A SO₄	30 mg	3 mo.	alcohol
		M	35	dl-A SO₄; d-A SO₄; meth-A HCl	250 mg	6 yr.	alcohol; bromides
		M	31	d-A SO₄; meth-A HCl	60 mg	5 yr.	alcohol; bromides
		M	30	dl-A SO₄	?	1 yr.	alcohol
		31 cases No individual data given					
McConnell & McIlwaine (1961) U.K.	126	5 cases No individual data given					
McConnell (1963) U.K.	125	1 case No individual data given					
Rickman, et al. (1961) U.S.A.	150	18 cases No individual data given for 15 cases					
		F	36	d-A SO₄	20 mg	1.5 yr.	coffee
		F	37	dl-A resin complex	60 mg	1 mo.	
		F	37	d-A SO₄	15 mg	2 mo.	
Young, et al. (1961) U.S.A.	201	M	12	d-A SO₄	20 mg	2 yr. +	
Grantham, et al. (1962) Canada	76	F	37	amphetamine	?	months	
		F	28	d-A SO₄	80 mg	?	
		M	40	amphetamine; thyroid	20 tablets	?	
		M	25	d-A SO₄	handfuls	?	
Kiloh & Brandon (1962) U.K.	109	12 cases No individual data given					
McCormick (1962) U.S.A.	127	M	58	meth-A HCl	20 mg (parenteral)	months	morphine
		M	59	dl-A SO₄; d-A SO₄	?	years	alcohol; barbiturates
		F	29	d-A SO₄; prochlorperazine	?	?	
		M	36	d-A SO₄	?	?	

*d-A SO₄—d-amphetamine sulfate
dl-A—amphetamine base
dl-A SO₄—amphetamine sulfate
meth-A—methamphetamine base
meth-A HCl—methamphetamine hydrochloride

Table IX. The remaining 7 cases did not fit this picture, 3 being instances of an amphetamine withdrawal psychosis, and will be described separately.

Table IX clearly indicates that the major mental symptoms were delusions of persecution present in 83 per cent of the cases and hallucinations of various kinds present in 63 per cent of the patients. Connell found paranoidal delusions in 81 per cent of his patients and his figures compare well with those of the present series with respect to the frequency of different types of hallucinations. Thus, in the present series there were visual hallucinations in 54 per cent of the cases, auditory hallucinations in 40 per cent, somatic or tactile hallucinations in 12 per cent, and olfactory hallucinations in 6 per cent. Connell's figures are 50, 69, 12, and 9 per cent respectively. Ideas of reference were present in 19 per cent of this series and in 59 per cent of Connell's group. This discrepancy may well be a matter of terminology rather than of substance, however. As Connell has emphasized, disorientation is rare in this condition since in both series it was present in only 7 per cent of the patients. Other mental symptoms found in these patients were hyperactivity or excitation (41 per cent), anxiety (26 per cent), hostility or aggressiveness (22 per cent), agitation (17 per cent), and depression (15 per cent). Thus, the mental condition during the psychotic episode in the majority of these cases is essentially the same as that described by Connell and consists, in his words, of "primarily a paranoid psychosis with ideas of reference, delusions of persecution, auditory and visual hallucinations, in a setting of clear consciousness."

In the 7 cases reported in which the clinical picture was less sharply delineated, it was nevertheless characterized by confused, delirious, hallucinated, or apparently schizophrenic states. Four of these occurred during chronic drug ingestion and 3 as withdrawal reactions following chronic intake. Brief descriptions of these cases follow.

Brown (32) reported the case of a sailor with a history of amphetamine use, who injured himself by jumping through the glass of a ticket office window after consuming the contents of 5 amphetamine inhalers during 48 hours while going without food or sleep. After recovery he could not recall the incident.

Peterson and Somerville (142) reported the case of a 29-year-old man with a history of psychopathy and drug addiction, including habitual consumption of 125–250 mg of amphetamine daily, who was certified as insane. On admission he showed mental retardation, foolish irrelevant talk, and detachment from his surroundings. Withdrawal symptoms were wakefulness, depression, headache, and hunger, but no craving. The provisional diagnosis was psychopathy with schizoid tendencies. Abely, et al. (1), reported two cases. A 29-year-old woman, who had been in the habit of consuming large quantities of d-amphetamine tartrate and phenmetrazine for years, presented with gross thought disturbances, lack of precision and flight of memories, inappropriate laughter, stereotypy, repetition of questions and words, inability to concentrate, incipient catatonia, gross delirium, and delusions and hallucinations. Although she had been diagnosed as a schizophrenic 2 years earlier she recovered after 3 months of treatment. The other was the case of a 19-year-old girl who had been consuming undetermined quantities of d-amphetamine tartrate and phenmetrazine for 2 years. She was admitted to hospital in a state of agitated confusion which cleared after 15 days.

The 3 cases of psychotic reactions following withdrawal of amphetamines were reported by Nandelstadh (132), Beamish and Kiloh (21), and Young, et al. (201). Nandelstadh describes the case of a 45-year-old man who suffered from acute confusional states on two occasions following withdrawal of amphetamine after prolonged periods of abuse of the drug. The confusion states appeared 2 weeks and 10 days after withdrawal respectively. Case 7 of Beamish and Kiloh was that of a 36-year-old man who had been consuming up to 25 capsules of Desbutal (d-amphetamine, 5 mg and Pentobarbital, 30 mg) daily for several years and who developed a confused and hallucinated state 3 days after withdrawal. The authors considered that the symptoms, which lasted for several days, may have been due to the withdrawal of the barbiturate. The third case, reported by Young, et al. (201), was that of a 12-year-old boy who had been taking 20 mg of d-amphetamine sulfate per day for over 2 years for the treatment of a hyperkinetic state. Because of insomnia the therapy was withdrawn and 14 days later he developed paranoid and somatic

TABLE IX

MENTAL SYMPTOMS IN CASES OF PSYCHOSIS ASSOCIATED WITH CHRONIC USE OF AMPHETAMINES

Author	Dis-orientation	Ideas of reference	Delusions of per-secution	Hallucinations and/or illusions — Auditory	Visual	Tactile	Olfactory	Depres-sion	Anxiety, fear, & terror	Agita-tion	Hos-tility	Hyper-activity	Duration after withdrawal	Relapses
Young & Scoville		x	x		x			x	x			x	5 wk.	
		x	x	x									more than 1 year	
Greving			x	x									12 days	
													10 days	
Staehelin			x	x				x	x			x	short	4
Daube		x	x										short	
		x	x	x									short	
		x	x	x		x	x			x		x	short	
		x	x	x			x		x		x		gradual recovery	1
Hartmann		x	x	x	x		x		x		x		6 wk.	
Norman & Shea		x	x	x	x	x			x	x	x	x	4 wk.	
Shorvon								x		x		x	short	
Hagenau & Aubrun				x		x							drug not withdrawn	
Harder		x	x	x					x	x		x	gradual recovery	
				x									gradual recovery	
Hernandez & Dalmau	x	x	x	x								x	1.5 days	
Schneck			x	x	x				x				2 days	
Brown			x	x	x				x	x			?	
													3 wk.	1
Freyhan			x					x	x	x			?	

TABLE IX (cont.)

Author	Dis-orientation	Ideas of reference	Delusions of persecution	Auditory	Visual	Tactile	Olfactory	Depression	Anxiety, fear, & terror	Agitation	Hostility	Hyperactivity	Duration after withdrawal	Relapses
Heuyer & Lebovici			x	x									3 days	
				x									?	
O'Flanagan & Taylor			x									x	1 wk.	18
Nandelstadh			x			x						x	3 days	
													?	
Knapp			x								x		?	
Alliez			x	x	?						x	x	3 wk.	1
Baruk & Joubert			x	x	x					x			?	
Pottier, et al.			x	x	x		x	x				x	5 mo.	
Bonhoff & Lewrenz			x	x	x				x			x	3 days	1
			x	x	x				x				3 days	
			x		x	x							2 days	
Carr				x	x				x		x	x	7 days	1
Chapman			x	x	x								6 wk.	
			x										more than 2 mo.	
Delay, et al.	x		x	x	x			x					more than 2 mo.	
	x												2 years	
			x	x					x	x	x	x	more than 1 year	
Herman & Nagler			x	x	x								?	
			x	x	x	x							prolonged	
			x	x	x	x							32 days	
			x	x	x								1 day	
Schinko			x	x	x			x	x			x	more than 7 wk.	

TABLE IX (cont.)

Author	Dis-orientation	Ideas of reference	Delusions of persecution	Hallucinations and/or illusions				Depression	Anxiety, fear, & terror	Agitation	Hostility	Hyperactivity	Duration after withdrawal	Relapses
				Auditory	Visual	Tactile	Olfactory							
Martimor, et al.			x		x	x						x	4 days	
Simpson					x				x		x		6 wk.	
Tolentino & D'Avossa			x	x	x	x						x	prolonged	
			x		x						x	x	?	
			x					x					?	
			x	x	x	x			x				?	1
			x	x	x	x			x		x	x	5 days	1
			x								x	x	1 yr.	
Wallis			x	x	x		x		x				days	1
Grahn			x								x	x	?	
Tolentino			x	x	x				x				?	
			x		x						x	x	6 days	
Askevold	x		x	x			x				x	x	3 days	1
			x							x	x	x	2 wk.	1
			x							x		x	weeks	
			x								x	x	14 days	
			x								x	x	14 days	
			x	x	x						x	x	7 days	
									x		x	x	?	
Fischer		x		x	x				x	x	x	x	12 days	
Beamish & Kiloh			x	x	x						x		weeks	9
		x	x	x	x				x		x		short	4
			x	x				x			x	x	days	1
											x		?	1
Ferrero	x		x		x					x	x	x	3 days	
											x	x	15 days	1

TABLE IX (concld.)

Author	Dis-orientation	Ideas of reference	Delusions of persecution	Auditory	Visual	Tactile	Olfactory	Depression	Anxiety, fear, & terror	Agitation	Hostility	Hyperactivity	Duration after withdrawal	Relapses
Marley	x	x	x					x		x		x	days	
		x		x	x						x	x	8 days	
		x											?	
	x	x	x	x	x			x				x	3 wk.	
		x	x	x	x			x		x			2 wk.	
Rickman, *et al.*			x	x	x			x	x				2 wk.	
		x	x										12 days	
			x									x	12 days	
Grantham, *et al.*			x	x	x	x			x		x		?	
			x	x									?	1
			x		x								?	
			x	x	x	x					x	x	?	1
McCormick			x	x	x								?	
			x		x								?	
					x								?	
			x		x		x						?	20
TOTALS FOR 87 CASES	6	12	72	35	46	10	5	13	23	15	19	36		

delusions, visual hallucinations, insomnia, impulsive unpredictable behavior, suspiciousness, and disorientation with respect to time. Later he became withdrawn, mute, and assumed bizarre positions. He then became cataleptic, had a mask-like facies, and was incontinent. He improved gradually and was discharged after 2 weeks. Askevold (14) also states that 4 of his series of 7 cases developed a delirium psychosis after withdrawal of amphetamines.

A detailed assessment of the mental condition during the psychotic episode of the 78 cases that have recently been reported collectively rather than individually is, of course, not possible. However, the information given in these reports generally appears to be in agreement with that examined so far. Thus, Marley (119), in a study of the signs of intoxication with stimulants of the amphetamine type (including phenmetrazine), found excessive activity both at rest and in motion in 8 out of 10 patients. Only 2 of the 10 cases could be considered as acute intoxications (phenmetrazine) of 3 and 7 days duration respectively. In the other 8 patients the drugs had been taken for periods of 2 months to 10 years. There was logorrhea with ideas of reference in 9 cases, paranoid material in 7, impaired attention and concentration in 7, visual and auditory hallucinations in 5, depressive features in 4, and suicidal ideas, ideas of influence, illusions, and impaired memory for recent events in 2 cases each. Diminished insight was common.

Hampton (85), reporting on a group of 31 cases of psychiatric conditions associated with the abuse of amphetamines, states that "although all of the patients had some, if not strong, paranoid symptomatology on admission, only five were eventually diagnosed as paranoid schizophrenia and one as a paranoid condition."

McConnell and McIlwaine (126) and McConnell (125) reported that 6 cases of psychotic illness associated with amphetamine abuse were indistinguishable from paranoid schizophrenia. In all cases the most prominent feature was the presence of paranoid delusions. All patients were tense, evasive, and suspicious. There were disorders of thought (e.g., thought-blocking, illogicality), depression, ideas of reference, and auditory and visual hallucinations. All patients were oriented, but distractible, and had poor powers of attention and concentration.

Rickman, *et al.* (150), reporting on 18 of a total of 28 cases of acute toxic psychotic reactions directly related to the use of amphetamines which were seen over a period of 3 years, stated that the characteristic findings were depression, followed by marked suspiciousness. There was logorrhea in 12 patients, pronounced persecutory feelings in 6, visual hallucinations in 8, and auditory hallucinations in 2. Kiloh and Brandon (109) claimed that amphetamine psychosis is the most striking complication of amphetamine abuse and that it usually takes the form of a schizophrenic-like illness. Twelve cases of this type were seen at the Newcastle General Hospital over a period of 3 years.

Since the clinical condition is indistinguishable from paranoid schizophrenia and physical signs of amphetamine intoxication are not found invariably, the diagnosis of amphetamine psychosis has been based on the fact that the symptoms disappear in a matter of days or weeks after withdrawal. As Connell has stated, it would be much better to employ chemical tests for the presence of amphetamine-like substances in the urine. To date, however, most authors have based their diagnosis on the course of the illness after withdrawal of the drug.

Although all the cases discussed in this chapter are instances of a psychosis associated with chronic use of amphetamines, not all are, strictly speaking, unequivocal examples of amphetamine psychosis proper. For example, the 2 cases reported by Young and Scoville (200) are complicated by the fact that the patients were narcoleptics. Although the psychotic symptoms diminished after withdrawal of amphetamine, neither patient appears to have recovered fully. In the case reported by Hagenau and Aubrun (81) amphetamine was not withdrawn completely but a substantial reduction in dosage led to amelioration though not to disappearance of the symptoms. The case reported by Simpson (168) also showed marked amelioration of both physical and mental symptoms after withdrawal, but here the picture was complicated because the patient had taken tablets containing both methamphetamine and thyroid extract for several years.

It should be noted that many of the histories under review indicate that the patients abused at one time or another a variety of other drugs, most conspicuously alcohol and barbiturates but also opiates, cocaine, marihuana, and analgesics. It would appear futile to attempt an evaluation of the role these drugs might have played in the development of the psychoses since in many instances the histories are vague, particularly with respect to time. In addition, abusers of amphetamines, like drug addicts generally, are notoriously evasive about providing information of this type.

An important number of cases appear to be true schizophrenics in whom the drug either precipitated or exacerbated the psychotic picture but in whom withdrawal did not lead to recovery. Examples of this kind are Case 2 reported by Chapman (39), 3 cases by Delay, *et al.* (54), Case 2 of Herman and Nagler (92), Case 3 of Tolentino and D'Avossa (176), 3 cases of Bell and Trethowan (22).

In 1954 Delay, *et al.* (54), called attention to the difference between true toxic amphetamine psychosis and what they call pseudo-amphetamine psychosis, or schizophrenia co-existing with amphetamine abuse. In the former, withdrawal of the drug leads to rapid recovery; in the latter the condition becomes chronic despite withdrawal. They consider that in pseudo-amphetamine psychosis the drug is originally taken, and the dosage gradually increased, to combat progressive intellectual inefficiency which is a symptom of incipient schizophrenia. The following case histories are examples of pseudo-amphetamine psychosis.

CASE 1. Delay, *et al.* (54), reported the case of a 21-year-old woman who had taken *d*-amphetamine tartrate for 6 years and large doses of it for several months before admission, in order to cope with the demands of a piano career. Her symptoms increased gradually and consisted of insomnia, anorexia, loss of weight, and headaches. Some weeks before admission ideas of persecution appeared. When seen she was agitated, anxious, and disoriented, and had developed logorrhea and stammering. Withdrawal of *d*-amphetamine and administration of sedatives diminished the agitation and anxiety but not her thought disorder and incongruity of affect. She improved after insulin coma therapy, but was re-admitted a year later to another hospital despite abstinence from *d*-amphetamine.

CASE 2. In 1954 Chapman (39) described the case of a 39-year-old man who was admitted to hospital complaining that a number of persons were plotting against him. About 4 months earlier he had begun to take amphetamine daily in doses of up to 90 mg for the purpose of working very intensely. Two months before admission he began to develop an elaborate system of paranoid delusions. On admission he was suspicious, but talked freely about his persecutory ideas. His sensorium was clear and there were no hallucinations. The patient's pre-psychotic personality had a distinctly paranoid trend. Although earlier he had used alcohol excessively and had had one episode of delirium tremens with florid paranoid delusions, he had not drunk at all for a year prior to admission. After a 2-month period of observation and conservative treatment his condition remained unchanged. The author felt "that in this case amphetamine had been an important agent in precipitating a psychosis in a patient who was emotionally predisposed to paranoid thinking."

Although, for the reasons already given, it is not possible to ascertain exactly how many of the cases under discussion were instances of amphetamine psychosis proper, at least 109 appear to be clear examples of the condition. The following are representative case histories.

CASE 1. In 1941 Greving (78) reported the case of a 27-year-old chemist who was admitted to hospital 2.5 years after he started to take methamphetamine. The drug had been prescribed for weakness, fatigability, and other symptoms. Initially it produced great improvement in mood and capacity for work in doses of 18 mg per day, but tolerance soon developed and he raised the dose to an average of 180 mg daily (maximum dose 215). The initial beneficial effects were not maintained, but marked side effects, such as insomnia, weight loss, and palpitations appeared. He became inattentive, slow-thinking, restless, and irresponsible and could not continue working. When marked obsessive-compulsive phenomena and sensory illusions of various types developed he entered the hospital voluntarily. After 12 days of withdrawal the compulsions and illusions disappeared but the physical signs of sympathotonia persisted for 2 to 3 weeks. Eventually he made a complete recovery. Greving noted that the pre-toxic personality of the patient was psychopathic and probably contributed to the particular psychic symptoms during the period of intoxication.

CASE 2. Norman and Shea (134) in 1945 described the case of a 49-year-old lawyer who was admitted to hospital with somatic, visual, and auditory hallucinations of four months' duration. He had been taking amphetamine sulfate in steadily increasing doses for 6 years. The drug had originally been prescribed (40 mg per day) for fatigue but later he continued to use it without the consent of his doctor in doses of up to 250 mg daily. Amphetamine enabled him to give up the use of alcohol which he had been taking since age 17. He was also a heavy smoker and excessively fond of sweets. The first symptoms were insomnia and restlessness followed by persecutory delusions and hallucinations. He became so fearful, sleepless, and hyperactive that hospitalization was advised. On admission he was agitated, resistive, hallucinated, and deluded (refusing food for 6 days), but physical examination was essentially negative. He was oriented, but had no insight and protested violently against illegal commitment. After 4 weeks in hospital his insight was good and he was discharged as recovered with a diagnosis of psychosis due to drugs and other exogenous toxins. The authors suggest that the alcoholic and the drug addict show many psychogenic factors of early life that arrest emotional development at the oral erotic stage as evidenced in this patient by excessive smoking, love of sweets, drinking, choice of profession, talkativeness, and drug addiction. They also note that the acute symptoms were very similar to those of acute alcoholic psychosis.

CASE 3. In 1955 Martimor, *et al.* (120), reported the case of a 38-year-old doctor who was admitted to hospital with hallucinations and ideas of persecution, but aware that he was intoxicated with *d*-amphetamine tartrate. He had begun taking 20 mg of *d*-amphetamine tartrate some months earlier because of personal problems. He took the drug intravenously. At first, with doses of 50 mg daily there was hyperactivity, marked but not unpleasant insomnia interrupted by periods of deep, almost comatose sleep, disturbances of the personality, anorexia, loss of weight, and mydriasis. A few attempts to give up the drug at this time failed: "I needed my injections to regain my calm." Progressive increase in dosage to 500 mg per day was accompanied by the development of delusions of persecution and he became isolated, seclusive, and morbidly jealous. Despite a decrease in dosage to 200 mg per day his delusions persisted, and in addition visual hallucinations appeared. Voluntary abstinence for 48 hours abolished the symptoms but a single injection brought them back and this led to his hospitalization. After 4 days of drug withdrawal in hospital the hallucinations and delusions disappeared completely. The authors note that the absence of pre-existing paranoidal traits and the complete disappearance of symptoms on withdrawal indicate a primary toxic psychosis, and in cases like this they consider the prognosis good unless the patient resorts to the drug again.

CASE 4. In 1960 Beamish and Kiloh (21) reported the case of a 35-year-old married man who had been taking d-amphetamine for 2 years in doses of up to 300 mg per day. For the past 3 years he had become increasingly aggressive, solitary, jealous of his wife, and preoccupied with religious subjects. On admission he was very tense, talked about religious matters in a rambling and almost incoherent manner, and thought that a bearded fellow patient was John the Baptist. There was no clouding of consciousness. When his condition settled he was allowed out but his psychotic symptoms, including paranoid delusions,

58

re-appeared. This time they lasted about 36 hours but for the next 5 days he was depressed. Both on admission and during this relapse his urine gave a positive methyl orange test for amphetamine. The patient was well a year after discharge from hospital, although the diagnosis of paranoid schizophrenia had been seriously considered.

CASE 5. In 1961 Rickman *et al.* (150), described the case of a 36-year-old married woman with no history of mental illness or maladjustments. She had been taking 5 mg of *d*-amphetamine sporadically for a year and a half, and 20 mg daily plus 8 to 10 cups of coffee for the 6 weeks prior to admission. For about 6 days before admission she had become increasingly tense, apprehensive, and suspicious and later developed illusions and hallucinations. On admission she was frightened, withdrawn, suspicious, and depressed, with blunted and inappropriate affect. Her answers were irrelevant. She had paranoidal delusions and auditory hallucinations. The symptoms cleared in 2 weeks and a year later she was well.

Physical Condition

Because of the diverse nature of these reports it is not possible to make an objective appraisal of the physical condition of the patients during the psychotic episode. However, the over-all impression is that physical signs of amphetamine intoxication, if any, were far less dramatic than the mental symptoms. This is illustrated by the fact that in a substantial number of reports no reference is made to physical symptoms (95, 132, 110, 3, 20, 39, 92, 176, 185, and 127). Otherwise the most commonly mentioned symptoms were anorexia and weight loss, insomnia, and tremors, particularly of the hands. Remarkably few authors make any mention of the presence of signs of sympathetic overstimulation, presumably characteristic of amphetamine overdosage.

With respect to physical signs of intoxication referable to the central nervous system, Marley (119) found that enhancement of postural function with augmented limb tone and tendon reflexes was typical. Other signs included mydriasis with impaired pupillary response to light, tremor of the tongue and limbs, and facial twitching and tics. Perhaps Connell's statement "that there are no diagnostic signs of amphetamine intoxication" could be modified to the effect that in amphetamine psychosis there are not *always* physical signs of amphetamine intoxication, but that in many cases signs, such as anorexia and weight loss, increased postural tone, and mydriasis, are present and should be of help in the diagnosis.

Effects of Withdrawal

The most dramatic effect of withdrawal in these patients was, of course, the disappearance or at least the diminution of the acute psychotic symptoms for which they had been hospitalized in the first place. Untoward withdrawal symptoms were not mentioned at all in a substantial number of reports, and in the remainder the most commonly observed symptom was depression which was specifically mentioned in 18 cases. Bell and Trethowan (22) who presented a series of 14 cases observed deep depression in 4, moderate depression in 5, and mild and short-lived depression in 4. Danger of suicide was present in 3 of their patients. They further state that the physical symptoms of withdrawal were few and unimportant. Hampton (85) who presented a series of 31 cases observed no untoward withdrawal symptoms, except for irritability in some patients. These findings are in general agreement with Connell's observations.

The only important difference between the Connell series and the series under discussion is that in 7 of the latter, psychotic episodes were attributed to the withdrawal of amphetamines. Of the 4 cases of this type described by Askevold (14) 3 had psychotic episodes during the period of intoxication with amphetamines and presumably during the withdrawal stage as well. In the fourth case the psychosis occurred only during withdrawal. These cases are very difficult to evaluate because in two of the patients there was barbiturate in the serum on admission and in another there was the strong suspicion that the patient was being provided with drugs by a friend. As will be recalled, barbiturates were also implicated in the case described by Beamish and Kiloh (21). Thus the evidence does not seem unequivocal enough to permit any conclusions about the authenticity of psychotic episodes as amphetamine withdrawal phenomena.

Since the clinical characteristics of these psychotic episodes were different from those observed during amphetamine intoxication, even in the same patients, and from psychotic reactions due to withdrawal of other drugs such as opiates, alcohol, and barbiturates,

60

Askevold concluded that there was a characteristic amphetamine withdrawal psychosis. He characterized it thus: it consists of a delirium with confusion and hallucinations; there is little or no reduction in muscle strength; the activity is constant throughout the day and night; there are few or no vegetative symptoms, apart from insomnia; the time elapsed between the beginning of withdrawal and the appearance of the delirium is comparatively long (3–10 days); and the symptoms last longer than in other withdrawal psychoses. The only other authors to have claimed the existence of an amphetamine withdrawal psychosis have been Nandelstadh (132), and Young, Simson, and Frohman (201).

Treatment

Since the symptoms of amphetamine psychosis proper disappear quite rapidly following withdrawal, it is obvious that only symptomatic or supportive treatment is required, and that, as Connell and Hampton among others have recommended, attention should be focused on the underlying disabilities that led the patient to abuse the drugs in the first place. It is equally obvious that in other instances where amphetamine either precipitated or exacerbated schizophrenia, the treatment should be that which is currently in use for this condition. A number of authors have resorted, in the case of amphetamine psychosis proper, to such therapeutic procedures as electroshock or insulin shock but this appears to have been due mainly to uncertain or mistaken diagnosis on admission.

Follow-up

Except for the survey of Bell and Trethowan (22) no planned follow-up study appears to have been made. However, in at least 20 of the remaining cases in Table VIII the patients had had previous psychotic episodes of short duration, or relapses after they were seen for the first time. Case 3 of McCormick (127), for example, had been hospitalized 20 times between 1946 and 1955 because of severe paranoidal delusions and hallucinations associated with excessive use of alcohol, barbiturates, and amphetamines. The hallucinations appeared to be due mainly to the amphetamines and would disappear during drug withdrawal in hospital. In 1950 O'Flanagan and Taylor (135) reported another remarkable case of a 38-year-old man who had been admitted to hospital 16 times in 16 years. On all occasions but one there was wild excitement, confusion, distractability, and marked paranoid delusions. Once when he was admitted more than 7 days after ceasing ingestion of amphetamine there was extreme depression. On each occasion, admission had been preceded by ingestion of large doses of amphetamine, and the maniacal phase cleared in a week after withdrawal of the drug. After the last admission he remained free from psychotic symptoms for 6 months until he resorted to the drug again during a period of stress. Beamish and Kiloh (21) reported one patient who had had nine relapses, another who had had four, and two who had had one each. Other authors who have reported cases with one or more relapses are Staehelin (170), Daube (52), Brown (32), Bonhoff and Lewrenz (29), Tolentino and D'Avossa (176), Wallis (185), Askevold (14), Ferrero (61), Bell and Trethowan (22), Hampton (85), and Grantham, Martin, and Rouleau (76).

Bell and Trethowan (22) were able to follow-up 12 of their 14 patients for periods ranging from 5 months to 6.5 years. They observed recurrent psychotic states associated with continued amphetamine intake in 4 of these patients.

A unique case in the literature concerns a German physician who was the subject of a report first by Daube (52) in 1942, and again 12 years later by Bonhoff and Lewrenz (29). According to Daube this 56-year-old married doctor had been mentally sound except for episodes of bad temper and aggressiveness and the occasional intake or morphine and cocaine. He began to take methamphetamine regularly, 2 years prior to his first admission to hospital, because of the demands of his work and of extra war duties. At first he took 3 tablets (18 mg) daily, then switched to injections, and finally was sniffing 60 powdered tablets daily. Gross psychic changes, consisting of somatic hallucinations, extreme suspiciousness and hostility, paranoid delusions directed mainly against his wife, and marked agitation began 3 months before admission. In hospital the hallucinations and delusions cleared gradually, but the marked hostility and poor insight remained. Bonhoff and Lewrenz state that they saw this patient later during the same year when he was committed to hospital with the same symptoms. He improved gradually, absconded from hospital, and was subsequently followed as an out-patient. In June of 1942 he resumed the intake of methamphetamine and took barbiturates as well. He intermittently took large doses of the drug as a preliminary to the group practice of gross sexual deviations. Rapid deterioration was followed by an agitated depression and admission to a psychiatric hospital in 1944. After the war he resorted to the abuse of sedatives and this led to an acute drug delirium with cardiac arryhthmia due to gross abuse of cardiac glycosides. At 65 he gave an impression of complete depravity and degeneration, and he had no insight at all, attempting to explain his previous hospitalizations as frame-ups by jealous colleagues.

It is apparent from these cases that the prognosis of amphetamine psychosis is bad in the sense that a patient who has once reacted in this way will repeatedly do so if he persists in continued abuse of the drug. Thus the prognosis is intimately related to his compulsive need for amphetamines and/or other drugs.

Age

The average age of 105 patients was 35 years with a range of 19 to 56 years. In the Connell series the average age was 32 years, 6 months, and the range 20 to 49 years. Only 12.5 per cent of Connell's patients and only 19 per cent of this group were over 40 years old. Other cases, reported in groups and not included in the averages above, would tend to confirm that amphetamine psychosis is more commonly seen in people in their 'twenties and 'thirties. Thus, the age range of 5 patients included in the report by McConnell and McIlwaine (126) was 22 to 46 years and in the series of 18 patients reported by Rickman, et al. (150), it was 20 to 39 years.

Sex

Of Connell's patients 64 per cent were men and 36 per cent women, compared to 60 per cent men and 40 per cent women in the series under consideration. However, of the 58 cases reported before 1958, 83 per cent were men as opposed to 47 per cent amongst the 105 cases reported since 1958. These figures suggest that the incidence of amphetamine psychosis among women has been increasing in recent years. In this respect it is interesting to note that as late as 1954, Herman and Nagler (92) believed theirs to have been the first case reported in the literature of amphetamine psychosis in a woman. In fact, at least 6 cases had been reported prior to 1954, 4 in France (81, 3, & 54), one in Germany (52), and one in the United States (110). In more recent years a few authors have noted that the condition appears to have become a more serious problem among women.

In 1960 Abely, *et al.* (1), presented 4 case reports of toxic psychosis in women associated with the abuse of phenmetrazine or a combination of phenmetrazine and amphetamines and stated that several cases of this type were seen during a one-year period. The patients were usually young female students or career women highly concerned with their appearance and originally resorting to these drugs for weight-control purposes. In 1961 Hampton (85) reported 31 cases of psychiatric conditions associated with abuse of amphetamines, of which 17 were women and 14 men, and expressed the opinion that people in medical and paramedical occupations and obese women with depressive tendencies are particularly susceptible to abuse of amphetamines. In an important study made by Kiloh and Brandon in 1962 (109) on various aspects of the consumption of amphetamines in Newcastle-upon-Tyne, the conclusion was drawn that amphetamine psychosis is the most striking psychiatric complication of amphetamine abuse and that the condition is more commonly seen in neurotic, easily depressed women. Other recent reports emphasizing the higher incidence of the condition among women are those of Rickman, *et al.* (150), from the United States, Grantham, *et al.* (76), from Canada, and McConnell and McIlwaine (126) and McConnell (125) from Northern Ireland.

Although the data available to date are not sufficient to explain the increasing frequency of amphetamine psychosis in women, it is possible that the phenomenon is related to the increasing concern among women with the problems of overweight, and to the broad use of amphetamines and allied drugs as anorectics. If large numbers of women resort to these drugs to lose weight it is not surprising that a certain proportion should become dependent on them, and that some of these would go on to develop psychosis.

Marital Status

Of 100 cases where the marital status was mentioned, 32 were single, 49 married, 8 separated, and 11 divorced. These figures do not agree very well with those of the Connell series where 50 per cent of the patients were single, 31 per cent married, and 12 per cent separated or divorced. A further inconsistency in this respect is illustrated by the report of Bell and Trethowan (22 & 23) where, of a total of 14 cases, one was married, 4 were single, and the rest were separated, divorced, and so forth. It is therefore not possible to draw any conclusions regarding the marital status of these patients which might presumably be taken as an index of their emotional maturity.

Occupation

Connell found that all walks of life and occupations were represented in his series. Unfortunately, information in this respect was given for only 69 patients in the present series. This small number, as well as the fact that these cases have been drawn from many different countries with different cultures and customs, makes it difficult to draw any valid generalizations. It is worth noting, however, that people in the medical and paramedical professions, and, in recent years, married women or housewives, are highly represented. Of the 69 patients, 30 (43 per cent) belonged to the medical or paramedical professions or were closely associated with people in these professions: 19 physicians, 2 pharmacists, 2 nurses, 1 medical student, 1 student midwife, 1 drug salesman, 1 chemist, and 3 wives of physicians. This is probably a fictitiously high proportion because this type of profession is more likely to be stated in a case history dealing with drug abuse than are other types. The other interesting point is that 17 of the 69 patients were housewives and that most of the reports concerning them have appeared in the literature since 1960. These figures are too scanty and their statistical significance too unreliable to be taken as true indexes of incidence of amphetamine psychosis in different occupations, but they may be useful to point the way for further surveys.

Amphetamines are reputedly widely used by university students in many countries at examination time and by long-haul truck drivers on this continent. It is therefore worthy of note that only 2 students were represented in this series and not a single truck driver. A probable explanation is that both students and truck drivers use these drugs only intermittently to keep awake during the performance of specific tasks, rather than chronically to counteract personality problems. Another factor with respect to students is that, though they may learn to use the drugs while at school or university, they may not develop drug dependence and toxic effects until later.

Original Reason for Taking Amphetamines, Duration of the Use or Abuse, Drugs, and Dosage

Of 93 cases in which the original reason for taking amphetamines is stated, 30 took it for weight-reducing purposes, 20 for depression, 16 as a substitute for alcohol or other drugs of addiction, 9 to combat feelings of fatigue, 7 to perform extra work, 7 to study, and 4 for narcolepsy. Thus, about a third of the patients originally took the drug for the control of obesity, and of these the majority were women. As has already been pointed out, most of these cases were described as recently as 1961, and 23 of them were reported by only 2 authors.

From the point of view of the prophylaxis of amphetamine psychosis it would be useful to be able to ascertain the proportions of cases in which the drug was prescribed by a physician, and of those in which it was self-administered. Reasonably unambiguous statements in this respect were found in only 61 cases. In 13 of these the drug was originally prescribed; in 48 it was self-administered. In the Connell series about a third of the patients for whom information was available had had the drug prescribed originally. These figures are too incomplete to allow any valid generalization with respect to the responsibility of the medical profession in introducing these drugs to potential abusers. However, it should be pointed out that one of the major current medical uses of amphetamines and allied drugs is for the treatment of obese patients, and that recent reports suggest a significant incidence of dependency to these drugs and of psychotic reactions in these patients.

The drugs taken, maximum daily doses, and duration of use are listed in Table VIII. In 73 of the 172 cases (excluding the Connell series) the drugs are referred to simply as amphetamines, and are stated to have been consumed in maximum daily doses ranging from 50 to 500 mg. Table X lists the specific drugs used in the remaining 99 cases and the range of maximum daily dose reported. It will be seen that the most commonly used drugs have

TABLE X

PREPARATIONS AND DOSE RANGES REPORTED IN CASES OF CHRONIC
AMPHETAMINE ABUSE WITH PSYCHOSIS

Drug	No. of cases	Range of maximum daily dose
Amphetamine sulfate	22	30–750 mg
Methamphetamine HCl	17	20–270 mg
d-amphetamine sulfate	15	15–350 mg
Amphetamine base	13	250–1250 mg
d-amphetamine tartrate	7	416–800 mg
Methamphetamine base	2	1250 mg
Methamphetamine tartrate	1	150 mg
Amphetamine resin complex	1	60 mg
Various amphetamines	21	30–1000 mg

been amphetamine sulfate and d-amphetamine, either as the sulfate or as the tartrate. Reports of amphetamine psychosis due to the abuse of methamphetamine hydrochloride have come principally from Germany and Italy. The figures clearly show that any of these drugs is potentially capable of producing a psychotic reaction. This point is of some interest because the literature has sometimes implied that not all amphetamines carry this risk. Worse still, individuals who take these drugs on their own initiative are often misled by new names given to various salts and mixtures. An interesting example of this kind reported by Tolentino (175) is that of a pharmacist who, in order to avoid habituation and toxic effects, varied his intake by selecting alternately from among such preparations as Desoxyn, Methedrina, Simpamina D, Pervitin, Psychergina, Psychodin, Simpoitina, all of which, unknown to him, are varieties of amphetamine. He developed a paranoid psychosis despite these precautions. Further confusion has arisen more recently with the introduction of the new anorectics, such as phenmetrazine and diethylpropion, which have been claimed not to be amphetamines, but which, nevertheless, have been shown to have generally the same actions and risks as the amphetamines proper.

The rather important question of the minimum dose of amphetamines capable of producing psychotic episodes when taken chronically is difficult to answer. The consensus among the authors is that these patients show a strong inclination to deny taking any drugs at all, or to minimize the dosage if confronted with the facts. Be this as it may, in several of the cases listed in Table VIII the maximum daily dose admitted was relatively small, that is 50 mg or less. These include: Case 8 of Askevold, 50 mg "amphetamine"; amphetamine sulfate, 30 mg in Case 1 of Chapman and 50 mg in Case 9 of Bell and Trethowan; d-amphetamine sulfate, 15 and 20 mg in Cases 3 and 1 respectively of Rickman, et al., 25 mg in Case 21 of Marley, and 30 mg in cases 19 of Marley and 11 of Bell and Trethowan; methamphetamine hydrochloride, 20 mg in Case 2 of McCormick and 30 mg in Case 3 of Tolentino and D'Avossa. This, in addition to the evidence already given in the chapter on acute toxicity, suggests that daily doses of 50 mg or less of amphetamines are able to produce psychotic reactions in certain individuals. However, it should be borne in mind that the accuracy of the information is often subject to question.

The largest doses stated to have been consumed were: "amphetamines," 500 mg (14); amphetamine base, 1250 mg (32); amphetamine sulfate, 750 mg (54); d-amphetamine sulfate, 350 mg (22); d-amphetamine tartrate, 800 mg (95); and methamphetamine hydrochloride, 270 mg (78). These figures presumably indicate the maximum daily doses tolerable, and taken together with the minimum doses capable of producing psychotic symptoms, they generally correspond to the known relative potencies of these drugs as central stimulants, that is d-amphetamine and methamphetamine are roughly twice as potent as racemic amphetamine. However, as will be shown later, some individuals can habitually consume equally large doses without developing psychotic symptoms.

A question intimately related to dosage is the duration of the abuse. This was specifically stated in 90 cases although, of course, all cases listed in Table VIII clearly implied chronic use. Twenty-five of the patients took the drugs for less than a year and of these 16 took it for less than 6 months. Of the remainder, 13 took it for 1 to 2 years, 9 for 2 to 3 years, 16 for 3 to 5 years, 16 for 5 to 10 years, 6 for an unspecified number of years, and only 6 for more than 10 years. These figures indicate wide variability in tolerance to the toxic effects of the drugs. More than half of the patients went on to develop a psychosis after a relatively short period of abuse of 2 years or less; a few were able to continue its use for more than 10 years.

In the vast majority of cases the drugs were taken orally, but in at least 7—(52), Cases 3 and 4; (29), Case 8; (3); (20); (120); (127), Case 2—they were taken by injection, mainly intravenously. In this respect, it is interesting to note that 4 of the latter patients were physicians and one a student midwife, and that at least 4 of them were or had been morphine addicts. Although the drug taken was amphetamine base in many of the cases, these patients did not inhale it but took it orally, either by chewing the contents of inhalers or by dissolving them in various beverages and swallowing the solutions. In at least one instance—(52), Case 4—methamphetamine hydrochloride was taken by sniffing up to 60 powdered tablets per day. This patient had occasionally taken not only morphine but cocaine as well.

Mental Background

Because certain individuals who consume amphetamines chronically in increasing amounts develop psychotic symptoms and others, as will be shown later, do not, the question arises of what, if anything, predisposes them to respond in this fashion. The points of view from which the histories included in this literature survey were written are so heterogeneous that they preclude a comprehensive answer to this interesting question.

One sign of abnormal behavior which is consistently referred to is the abuse of other drugs. At least 91 patients took alcohol or other drugs in excess at one time or another. Although this feature points out the proneness to drug dependence in these patients, it is of little relevance in explaining the development of psychotic symptoms, since many patients abuse amphetamines and/or other drugs without becoming psychotic. A number of recent reports by various authors, each including a reasonably large series of patients, illustrate the difficulties inherent in this problem.

In 1954 Herman and Nagler (92) described 8 patients suffering psychiatric disturbances associated with abuse of amphetamines, 4 of whom had taken the drug for a month or more. The authors state that 7 of the patients had psychopathic traits, such as promiscuity, lack of discipline, criminal behavior, poor work histories, and drug addiction. The eighth patient, who did not show psychopathic traits, suffered a neurotic episode of one week's duration.

Askevold (14) describes "personality traits," social status, and predisposing factors in the 7 patients of his series who suffered from amphetamine psychoses. Under "personality traits" he includes such attributes as extraversion, ambition, and activity. He states that 6 of the patients were of above average social status and one below average. Among "predisposing traits" he refers to alcoholism, and marital and work difficulties. He further states that of the other 7 patients of his series who abused amphetamines but did not develop paranoid episodes, 5 belonged to a lower social level and that their common personality characteristic was "weakness of character."

Beamish and Kiloh (21), who also presented a series of 7 cases, state that evidence of abnormal personality before the commencement of the drug abuse was common, and that in some the personality disorder appeared to be emphasized and aggravated by amphetamine, making social adaptation even more difficult. According to these authors all their patients showed evidence of a psychopathic personality. The incidence of other drug addictions was high and, as in the Askevold series, the social status of the patients, at least before the beginning of the period of drug abuse, also tended to be high.

In their series of 14 patients Bell and Trethowan (22 and 23) assessed what they called the psychosocial background of the patients in terms of family history, occupation, personality type, pre-existing sexual adjustment, and intelligence level. All patients

70

showed evidence of underlying personality instability such as neurotic or pre-psychotic traits, but no single or specific pattern of disturbance common to all. They had all had a disturbed childhood with a high incidence of alcoholism and mental illness in their family histories. The pre-existing sexual adjustment was poor, the series including cases of homosexuality, frigidity, and poorly adjusted heterosexuality. As opposed to the series presented by Askevold (14) and by Beamish and Kiloh (21) the social status of the patients, judging by their occupations, appeared to be low.

According to Hampton (85) all of his 31 patients had severe personality problems with depression playing a major part in 17. The psychiatric diagnoses after remission of the toxic state included 16 cases of schizophrenia, 8 with paranoid trends, 9 cases of psychopathic personality, 5 manic-depressive psychoses, and one psychoneurosis.

From this review it can be seen that different authors have used essentially different systems of classification in describing the pre-psychotic personalities of the patients. For example, Herman and Nagler and Beamish and Kiloh deal mainly with behavioral history, Askevold refers to personality types, while Hampton, and to some extent Bell and Trethowan, deal with clinical psychiatric diagnoses. The differences in the type of criteria employed in the earlier literature were reviewed by Connell (42). On the whole the commonest terms encountered are "psychopathic personality" and "personality defects." Reference to the numerous individual case histories, however, reveals that these terms are applied to the whole gamut of personality types ranging from irresponsible, ineffective, or withdrawn individuals through delinquents to aggressive, overambitious, hardworking married people with apparently normal social activities. Except for Connell, who considered that 6 of his patients had essentially normal personalities prior to the toxic state, few authors have made this claim. However, the diagnosis of mental *normality* would seem at best a most difficult problem, particularly because the authors in question belong to different schools of psychiatric thought, to different cultures, and to different times. Furthermore, it should be emphasized that in most cases these assessments were

71

made in retrospect, a factor which most likely prejudiced the appraisals.

This problem leads directly to the question of whether amphetamine produces true toxic psychoses or simply acts as a trigger in pre-psychotic individuals, especially those with latent paranoid traits. Young and Scoville (200), who were the first to describe psychoses associated with chronic use of amphetamines, were also the first authors to suggest that the drug precipitates a psychosis in patients with latent paranoid trends by making them more alert and observant, leading to ideas of reference and misinterpretations. Other authors to have expounded this view are Schneck (159), Freyhan (67), O'Flanagan and Taylor (135), Chapman (39), Simpson (168), and McCormick (127). Tolentino and D'Avossa (176) considered that, although this was not always the case, it was the most common, thus explaining why so many individuals do not react abnormally to large doses or prolonged use while a few became addicts and/or develop a psychosis.

Several authors, on the other hand, have emphasized the toxic role of the drug itself. Greving (78) felt that although the pre-toxic personality was a contributory factor, the mental symptoms during intoxication with high doses of methamphetamine were suggestive of mescaline action. Staehelin (170) called attention to the similarity between methamphetamine psychosis and the reactions produced by such other drugs as cocaine and khat. He considered the hallucinations to be largely related to sensory hyperacuity, and the delusions to be based partly on the pre-existing psychopathology and partly on a direct drug effect which impairs appraisal of reality by non-specific stimulation of sensation and associations. Hartmann (89) and Harder (87) compared the reactions to alcoholic hallucinosis and the latter stated that the absence of paranoidal ideas in the pre-psychotic stage indicated the importance of the exogenous as opposed to the constitutional factor. Martimor, et al. (120), presented one case in which the lack of pre-existing paranoidal traits and the complete disappearance of symptoms on withdrawal indicated a primary toxic effect. Yet in another of their cases an overt psychosis was precipitated by a single dose in a previously psychopathic patient.

72

Beamish and Kiloh (21) are also of the opinion that the evidence provides "little or no support for the view that in these cases an incipient or latent schizophrenia had been brought to light by amphetamine." Their conclusion was based on the following facts. (1) The course of the illness differs sharply from that of schizophrenia. (2) None of their 7 cases had schizophrenic relatives. (3) In one case a psychotic episode of the same kind was associated with a high dosage of bromide and chloral. However, they do not consider these paranoid states as specific effects of the amphetamines because many other agents give rise to similar pictures and amphetamines may sometimes give rise to other forms of psychosis. They offer the view that the symptoms may result from the products of abnormal adrenaline metabolism as has been suggested for schizophrenia by Hoffer and Osmond (96). Since many different processes can cause the same type of paranoid psychosis it could be regarded as the expression of a final common path, which in schizophrenia would be activated by a metabolic abnormality dependent partly on genetic structure.

The evidence presented in this review clearly shows that both views on the pathogenesis of psychosis associated with amphetamine consumption are correct and not mutually exclusive. Amphetamines can precipitate a chronic psychotic state in individuals with latent psychotic traits or aggravate overt symptoms of schizophrenia as has been shown by Liddell and Weil-Malherbe (118) for example. But the evidence is equally convincing that they can produce a transitory toxic psychosis in normal individuals or in patients with mental abnormalities of various types such as psychopaths, psychoneurotics, and manic depressives. In addition, it should be recalled that although a paranoid psychosis is the most common reaction, other types of psychotic pictures have also been described.

These conclusions are of considerable importance because they show clearly the impossibility of distinguishing *a priori* good from bad risks when prescribing these drugs. As Connell has pointed out, the notion quite prevalent in the literature and among general practitioners that only psychopaths, or only potential schizophrenics, are likely to abuse amphetamines and go on to develop a psychotic state should be discarded. Since the drugs can produce these reactions in individuals with all sorts of mental and emotional make-ups after either a single dose or during chronic abuse, the risks would appear to be great. This conclusion has often been challenged on the grounds that the condition is rare, considering the widespread use of these drugs. The discussion that follows will show that the true incidence of the condition is not known and that what little evidence there is points to the contrary.

Incidence of Amphetamine Psychosis

In several of the histories under discussion, reference is made to the effect that the patients had had previous psychotic reactions which had been diagnosed as schizophrenia and in which the role played by the use of amphetamines was not understood. The evidence collected here raises but does not answer the question of the true incidence of amphetamine psychosis or of a psychosis exacerbated by amphetamine abuse. The information available, however, and especially the increase in the number of reports since the publication of the Connell monograph in 1958, strongly suggests that the condition is far more frequent than it is believed to be. The real problem is the proper diagnosis of the condition; this would require full awareness on the part of the psychiatric profession of the existence and characteristics of this type of toxic psychosis.

The correct diagnosis of amphetamine psychosis is important with respect to treatment and prognosis. As noted earlier the psychosis, as opposed to true schizophrenia, requires no special treatment except for withdrawal of the drug. In these cases, as Connell noted, it is the underlying continued dependence on amphetamines and the concomitant personality disorders that require treatment. It is obvious, therefore, that if the condition is mistakenly diagnosed as schizophrenia the treatment will be inappropriate and the patients will return to their drugs and suffer from recurrent psychotic reactions and other disabilities.

Of the cases listed in Table VIII, 71 were reported from the United States, 64 from the United Kingdom, 16 from Australia, 12 from France, 11 from Germany, 9 from Italy, 7 from Norway, 4 from Canada, 2 from Switzerland, and 1 each from Austria and Argentina.

It is significant that the 4 cases reported from Canada were described as recently as 1962 (76), in a paper in which it is further stated that, between 1956 and 1960, 24 other cases of amphetamine intoxication (21 women and 3 men) were seen at the Roy-Rousseau Clinic in Quebec City, and 11 cases at the Department of Psychiatry of Laval University. Since it is most unlikely that amphetamine abuse in Canada is peculiar only to the city of Quebec, the probabilities are that the lack of reports from other centers is due either to a lack of recognition of the condition or to a failure to report cases of this type. Failure to report such cases in the literature undoubtedly occurs. However, the evidence presented here strongly suggests that lack of recognition of amphetamine psychosis is probably more frequent and unquestionably more serious from the point of view of public health.

Informal inquiries at the Ontario Hospital (Toronto) and at the Toronto Psychiatric Hospital revealed that although some cases of amphetamine psychosis have been diagnosed in this city, a proper evaluation of the total number of cases would require a specific survey. It should be emphasized, however, that without the appropriate facilities for chemical determination of amphetamines in the urine, the results of such a survey would be at best incomplete.

SUMMARY

The most serious and most frequently reported toxic effect of chronic amphetamine consumption is a psychotic reaction usually mistaken for schizophrenia. Though this condition was first reported in 1938, the most important and comprehensive assessment of it was a review of 42 original cases by Connell in 1958. A detailed review of the literature for the present study revealed 201 cases from all countries, including Connell's series, but excluding those reported in Japan.

By far the most common clinical picture is one of paranoid delusions and vivid hallucinations of all senses but without disorientation. Occasionally the patient is confused and violently excited. Usually the condition clears rapidly on withdrawal of the drug. However, in a small but appreciable number of cases the persistence of symptoms for a long time after drug withdrawal indicates that amphetamine may act as a precipitating factor in the onset of true schizophrenia. There are no diagnostic physical signs, the usual findings being those of sympathetic and central nervous overstimulation characteristic of the drug. The only important withdrawal symptoms are transitory but occasionally severe depression and lethargy. Treatment consists essentially of drug withdrawal, though many patients have received needless shock and other therapy because of mistaken diagnosis. Unless treatment is directed to the drug abuse rather than to the psychosis, the relapse rate is high.

Most of the patients are adults aged 20 to 50 years. Earlier reports indicated the majority of the patients were men, but in recent years the proportion of women has increased steadily. The two most numerous groups are people in the medical and paramedical professions, and obese housewives. Correspondingly the two commonest reasons for beginning the use of the drug are to improve mood and performance and to inhibit the appetite. All the amphetamines have been implicated, usually in doses well above the recommended therapeutic level. Most of the patients appear to have taken them without medical prescription. In most cases one to five years of chronic drug abuse preceded the onset of the psychosis. The majority of patients were described as psychopathic or neurotic, but their temperament and personalities varied widely and some were said to be normal before starting to use the drugs. There is, therefore, no characteristic mental or emotional picture by which a "high risk" patient can be identified in advance.

The frequency of reports of amphetamine psychosis has increased markedly since the appearance of Connell's monograph. A notable feature has been the number of large series reported by individual clinicians who have looked systematically for the condition. This suggests that the true incidence is much higher than has hitherto been appreciated and indicates the importance of routine chemical tests for amphetamines in schizophrenic patients.

76

V. Amphetamine Dependence, Habituation, and Addiction

ALTHOUGH A GREAT DEAL has been written about whether or not amphetamines are addictive drugs, there is as yet no consensus on this very important point. This has been due partly to lack of well-documented evidence, but to a far greater extent to the disagreement over what constitutes addiction. The crux of the disagreement has been whether or not amphetamines, when consumed chronically, produce physical dependence as manifested by the presence of clear-cut withdrawal symptoms and, therefore, strong craving. Thus, authors who have based their judgment almost exclusively on the question of physical dependence have argued that amphetamines do not produce addiction. Other authors, who have attached greater importance to such factors as compulsion to continue taking the drugs, development of tolerance, and harmful effects, have drawn the opposite conclusion.

Before going any further with the examination of this problem it should be pointed out that in the pertinent literature value judgments are clearly implicit, to the effect that addiction, if proven, would condemn these drugs as bad, whereas a verdict of habituation, dependence, or abuse would largely exonerate the drugs but condemn the *habitués*, dependents, or abusers. The discussion therefore seems to hinge on the identity of the culprit: the drug or its user. Also, the term "addiction," however defined, seems to carry with it the connotation of a very serious medical problem, while "habituation" is generally regarded, as has been recently pointed out by Connell (43), "in the same way as nail-biting, smoking, eating sweets, etc., and of being of little consequence."

In an attempt to resolve difficulties of this type, not only with respect to the amphetamines but to other drugs as well, the

World Health Organization Expert Committee on Addiction-Producing Drugs defined the terms drug addiction and drug habituation in 1950 (192) and 1952 (193) and revised these definitions as follows in 1957 (194):

Drug addiction is a state of periodic or chronic intoxication produced by the repeated consumption of a drug (natural or synthetic). Its characteristics include:
    (1) An overpowering desire or need (compulsion) to continue taking the drug and to obtain it by any means;
    (2) A tendency to increase the dose;
    (3) A psychic (psychological) and generally a physical dependence on the effects of the drug;
    (4) Detrimental effect on the individual and on society.

Drug habituation (habit) is a condition resulting from the repeated consumption of a drug. Its characteristics include:
    (1) A desire (but not a compulsion) to continue taking the drug for the sense of improved well-being which it engenders;
    (2) Little or no tendency to increase the dose;
    (3) Some degree of psychic dependence on the effect of the drug, but absence of physical dependence and hence of an abstinence syndrome;
    (4) Detrimental effects, if any, primarily on the individual.

The distinction between the two conditions was thus based on the following attributes: *compulsion* versus *desire* to continue taking the drug; *tendency* versus *little or no tendency* to increase the dose; psychic and *generally physical dependence* versus psychic but *no physical dependence* and therefore *absence of an abstinence syndrome*; detrimental effects *on the individual and on society* versus detrimental effects *on the individual*. Thus the presence of physical dependence, generally but not necessarily, and detrimental effects on society were the only qualitative differences between addiction and habituation established by these definitions.

In 1964 the Expert Committee (195) recognized that these definitions had failed, in practice, to establish a clear distinction between the two concepts and that, although the notion of addiction gained some acceptance, the term continued to be misused. The problem was further compounded by a large increase in the number and diversity of drugs subject to abuse. Since psychic and/or physical dependence appears to be the constant element in drug abuse generally, the Committee has now adopted the term "'drug dependence,' with a modifying phrase linking it to a particular drug type in order to differentiate one class of drugs from another." Drug dependence is defined "as a state arising from repeated administration of a drug on a periodic or continuous basis. Its characteristics will vary with the agent involved and this must be made clear by designating the particular type of drug dependence in each specific case—for example, drug dependence of morphine type, of cocaine type, of cannabis type, of barbiturate type, of amphetamine type, etc." The Expert Committee has recommended the substitution of the term "drug dependence" for the terms "drug addiction" and "drug habituation" and notes that it "carries no connotation of the degree of risk to public health or need for a particular type of drug control."

The Expert Committee has characterized "drug dependence of amphetamine type" as "a state arising from repeated administration of amphetamine or an agent with amphetamine-like effects on a periodic or continuous basis. Its characteristics include:

(1) A desire or need to continue taking the drug;
(2) Consumption of increasing amounts to obtain greater excitatory and euphoric effects or to combat fatigue, accompanied in some measure by the development of tolerance;
(3) A psychic dependence on the effects of the drug related to a subjective and individual appreciation of the drug's effects; and
(4) General absence of physical dependence so that there is no characteristic abstinence syndrome when the drug is discontinued.

The new approach of the Expert Committee to the general problem of drug abuse should be welcomed since it avoids a distinction between habituation and addiction and thus the rather futile arguments concerning the relative dangers and merits of many drugs. The more realistic view implied in the new recommendations, that the degree of dependence produced by drugs of very diverse nature involves a continuum rather than sharply delineated differences, should be helpful in the better understanding and handling of the general problem. Whether these new recommendations will be generally accepted remains, of course, to be seen. It is not unlikely that controversy will continue for some time, since the whole question of drug abuse, even at the medical and scientific levels, is riddled with moral and ethical implications. Connell (43), for example, has already regretted the introduction of the term "drug dependence" when he states: "Here, again, there is a watering down of the concept [of addiction] so far as the average family doctor is concerned."

In 1963 the Council on Drugs of the American Medical Association (46) had already decided to abandon the use of the terms habituation and addiction. They stated: "The Council has come to recognize that its continued use of these terms for nonnarcotic drugs may lead to misinterpretation by legislators, law-enforcement officials, and the laity, as well as by physicians. Therefore, the Council has determined to replace the terms 'habituation' and 'addiction' in its statements with descriptions of the characteristics reported, or considered likely, to occur." The type of misinterpretation and confusion referred to above is perhaps best illustrated by another statement from the Council on the same page (45), where it is pointed out that although there is no specific reference to "addiction" in the monographs on the amphetamines in the 1962 edition of *New and Nonofficial Drugs*, the monograph on phenmetrazine states: "Addiction to this drug has been reported and resembles that observed with administration of the amphetamines."

The literature on the amphetamines in particular contains many an example of the efforts spent by numerous authors in trying to fit the evidence into concepts of habituation or addiction. These efforts will become irrelevant if the new definitions are widely adopted. However, it is worth examining the evidence in terms of the older definitions, since the assessment of the seriousness of the problem by many writers appears to hinge upon their decision as to whether the amphetamines are addictive or merely habituating. Authors who have argued against the notion that the amphetamines produce addiction include the following.

Hagenau and Aubrun (81) described the case of a 52-year-old woman who had amphetamine sulfate prescribed at age 47 because of overwork and depression. At first, 5 mg per day gave her an unusual feeling of well-being, but some months later 50 mg per day was barely effective. A year later she was taking 700 mg daily in single doses of 50 mg. She tried to stop but could not because withdrawal led to fatigue and inability to concentrate or to make any effort. At 48 she began to have tactile and visual hallucinations which seriously affected her behavior. Examination revealed autonomic disturbances such as dyspnea, tachycardia, vasomotor instability, alternating hunger and anorexia, dryness of mouth, and tremors. Blood pressure was 190/90. There were no disturbances of sleep, and despite some degree of mental apathy her mood was stable. There was no indication of intellectual deterioration. She was unable to give up the drug completely but under supervision she reduced the intake substantially and this was accompanied by a diminution of the frequency and vividness of her hallucinations. The authors concluded that this was not a case of true addiction (*toxicomanie vraie*) with habituation, craving, reactive depression, perversion, and withdrawal symptoms.

In 1956 Röhl (153) surveyed the literature in the German language to assess the addiction liabilities of methamphetamine. He pointed out that this drug had been put on the narcotics lists in Germany in 1941 largely because of the opinion of Speer who predicted that the euphoriant action of the drug would produce a strong risk of addiction, especially in psychopaths. Röhl felt, however, that secondary amines such as methamphetamine often show significantly fewer toxic effects than the corresponding primary amines and that, therefore, the addictive liability of methamphetamine should be evaluated separately. According to him, of the 15 reports between the years 1940 and 1954 warning about the addictive risks of methamphetamine only 3 backed their contentions with original case histories. The rest gave only general opinions which he did not consider convincing evidence. Many of the reports dealt with mixed addictions and since meth-amphetamine has been reported to potentiate the action of morphine, antihistaminics, and other drugs he suggested that many cases might be examples of potentiation rather than of direct methamphetamine action. He noted that in the 19 cases of pure methamphetamine addiction reported, the patients began using the drug principally to increase endurance, in contrast to morphine addicts whose primary motive was the induction of euphoria. The statistics on pure methamphetamine addiction he considered scarce and unreliable, these cases constituting probably less than 0.05 per cent of the total mental clinic population. This was in contrast with the nearly 500 papers reporting excellent therapeutic results with virtually no risk of addiction. Röhl concluded that methamphetamine does not fulfil the World Health Organization definition of an addictive drug because it produces no withdrawal symptoms and no tolerance except in psychopaths, and that therefore the current legal restrictions in Germany were not justified.

Grahn (75) also concluded that addiction to the amphetamines was extremely rare. He considered that most so-called "amphetamine addicts" are instances of "symptomatic addiction," that is, a non-specific type of addiction where the patient uses a substitute when his favorite drug is not available. He concluded: "Long-term therapy in itself does not produce an addiction to the drugs. It appears, instead, that addiction or habituation to amphetamine is caused by a factor in the individual's psychologic make-up which leads him to abuse the drugs rather than by any pharmacologic action of the drugs themselves. For these reasons, it seems that amphetamine therapy may be used for long periods of time with a great deal of safety."

Stungo (171) considered that the World Health Organization definition of addiction did "not sufficiently emphasize the occurrence of abstinence symptoms on withdrawal of an addictive drug" which he felt was the "only real distinction between addiction and habituation." According to this criterion, addiction to the amphetamines rarely occurs since (according to Stungo) they produce no tolerance, "true compulsive craving," or withdrawal symptoms following even prolonged use. The depression and sleepiness seen "occasionally" after discontinuing amphetamine therapy were attributed to exhaustion following a prolonged period of overstimulation and "do not necessarily constitute evidence of physical dependence." According to Stungo the psychological make-up of the individual is paramount and the pharmacological action secondary, since withdrawal rarely produces serious discomfort and the patients are just as prone to become "addicted" to tea, coffee, or tobacco and very frequently resort to other drugs. Stungo concluded: "It can accordingly be categorically stated that addiction or habituation to amphetamine alone is extremely rare and that when it does occur the patient is suffering from a condition which is not specific to the amphetamines."

Professor Chauncey D. Leake's *The Amphetamines—Their Actions and Uses* (116) contains many statements to the effect that the drugs are both extremely useful in medical practice and free of toxic effects and other untoward consequences such as addiction. A few quotations follow:

There are few clinical reports of toxic reactions in single or repeated doses of the amphetamines in man, except in unusual cases reported by Japanese workers (p. 30).

Long continued administration of ordinary doses of the amphetamines at appropriate intervals is remarkably free of any indication of undesired effect. There is little tolerance, and there is no clear evidence of addiction in the sense that there is craving or physical dependence (p. 30).

In the meanings defined here [according to the W.H.O. definitions], the amphetamines are not truly addictive drugs, although tolerance to them may develop, and an individual may become habituated to their use (p. 110).

The difference between morphine and alcohol, as common addiction drugs on the one hand, and the amphetamines on the other hand, is simply that the continued and repeated use of amphetamines does not involve withdrawal symptoms when these drugs are stopped, nor do the amphetamines produce a significant craving for the drugs themselves (p. 111).

Occasional claims of addiction to amphetamine sulfate have been made. These are not satisfactorily substantiated (p. 112).

No clear case of addiction to d-amphetamine has been reported (p. 113).

It is remarkable that in spite of occasional newspaper stories of addiction to "pep pills" or to abuse of Benzedrine inhalers, or to abuse of amphetamine administration by truck drivers, no specific case histories with clinical data for any such instance appear to have been reported (p. 114).

And finally,

> The over-all use of the amphetamines under medical direction has been helpful in a great variety of clinical conditions, and the abuses have been relatively insignificant and inconsequential. All the evidence indicates that the amphetamines are valuable and useful drugs in a wide variety of clinical conditions, and that under the circumstances of their use by millions of people, the occasional reports of possible habituation, or untoward reaction are extremely insignificant (p. 123).

These examples show that the major argument used against the notion that amphetamines are addictive drugs is the lack of physical dependence after prolonged use and therefore of a characteristic withdrawal syndrome. But in addition, emphasis has been put on the scarcity of reports, on the fact that many amphetamine abusers are or have been addicted to other drugs as well, and on the pathological personalities of the individuals involved.

Recent authors who have emphasized the seriousness of the question of chronic amphetamine abuse, whether it be called addiction, habituation, or dependence, are Connell (42 & 43), Bell and Trethowan (22 & 23), McCormick (127), Kiloh and Brandon (109), and Oswald and Thacore (137), among others.

In his *Amphetamine Psychosis* Connell (42) used the term "addiction" throughout the text. In a more recent publication entitled "Amphetamine Misuse" (43), he reviews the various definitions of the terms habituation and addiction by the World Health Organization and by the Interdepartmental Committee on Drug Addiction in Britain in 1961 and concludes: "The Interdepartmental Committee, in my view, erred in going back to the old views about addiction and limiting this to drugs which produce physical dependence and an abstinence syndrome. The merit of the 1950 W.H.O. definition was that under a label of addiction— a label which all take seriously—certain drugs such as the amphetamines could be considered seriously. Now, we are asked to consider them merely as drugs of habituation." After stressing that in amphetamine abuse "there may be a tendency to increase the dose and that detrimental effects upon society as well as upon the individual can occur," Connell adds: "The definitions given by the Committee are, in my view, too precise and arbitrary and fail to allow for a continuum between habituation and addiction in which an individual may begin by being habituated and then progress gradually along the path which leads to craving, increased dose taking and addiction."

Bell and Trethowan in a paper entitled "Amphetamine Addiction" (22) concluded: "Despite the widespread use of amphetamine for therapeutic and other purposes, review of the literature reveals some controversy as to whether addiction actually does occur, and contradictory views as to its frequency. Detailed study of 14 cases led the authors to the conclusion that amphetamine addiction is a definite and not uncommon entity."

McCormick (127), in a report which included 6 original cases of toxic reactions to amphetamine, stated: "Through the literature there is a constant harangue whether the amphetamines are truly addicting. There are those who argue that physical dependence on amphetamines is not acquired even by the heavy user and that patients may tend to become 'habituated' to the drug or may 'abuse' the drug, but they do not become 'addicted' to it. There is also considerable discussion about the diagnosis of addiction, especially with reference to the W.H.O. definition. Few users of amphetamines are found to fit that definition. I do not wish to enter the argument of addiction, habituation, or abuse—for the most part it is a matter of semantics. The important fact is that amphetamines can cause reactions that result in, or amplify, a psychiatric illness, whether the patient be addicted, habituated or just abusing the drug."

In an important study on the incidence of amphetamine abuse in Newcastle-upon-Tyne, Kiloh and Brandon (109) concluded in 1962: "It must be conceded that a number of patients taking excessive quantities of amphetamine fulfil this definition [of addiction according to the W.H.O.]. They certainly suffer an overpowering desire to continue taking the drug, they take it in amounts far exceeding the usual therapeutic dose, they may be prepared to break the law to obtain supplies, they are dependent upon it, and they sometimes become psychotic. Furthermore, withdrawal symptoms may occur, notably states of depression in which suicide may occur. Nevertheless, in the majority it would be more reasonable to regard these patients as habituated rather than addicted, though the distinction is only a quantitative one and largely a matter of definition."

Oswald and Thacore (137) demonstrated in 1963 that withdrawal of amphetamine or phenmetrazine in 6 women addicts led to physical abnormalities of nocturnal sleep patterns which disappeared immediately if the drugs were re-administered, or in three to eight weeks if the drugs were withheld. The authors concluded that amphetamine and phenmetrazine are truly addictive drugs since "*physical dependence* and characteristic, persisting, and easily measurable 'physical' or physiological abnormalities form part of the *abstinence syndrome*." With respect to the other characteristics of addiction as applied to amphetamine these authors stated: "Up to 10 times the 'therapeutic' dose is common among amphetamine and phenmetrazine addicts. These preparations produce a detrimental effect on the individual and on society. In the former they produce an egocentricity of outlook and impairment of those skills necessary to the conduct of successful social relationships, sometimes physical harm, and occasionally a frank psychosis. In paying for the pill, addicts sometimes acquire appalling financial debts. In society, the drugs encourage shady trafficking. Persons taking these drugs certainly experience an intense craving to continue so to take them by almost any means—these means, it is admitted, are not pursued to the extremes found, for instance, among morphine addicts. Extreme behavior is unnecessary with the laxity of current controls. We have demonstrated physical dependence can exist."

Still other authors such as Knapp (110) and Zondek (202) have taken intermediate positions. Knapp, after a thorough examination of 14 cases of amphetamine abuse, came to the conclusion that: "In short, using a broad concept of addiction,* we can say that addiction to amphetamine does occur. It is not accompanied by

---

*"Addiction is a state of periodic or chronic intoxication, detrimental to the individual and to society, produced by the repeated administration of a drug. Its characteristics are a compulsion to continue taking the drug and to increase the dose, with the development of psychic, and sometimes physical dependence on the drug's effects. Finally, the development of means to continue the administration of the drug becomes an important motive in the addict's existence." Definition of the Drug Addiction Committee of the National Research Council (98a).

marked physical dependence, or disabling physical consequences. Various addicts have used it in combination with other drugs. While taking it some unstable personalities have broken down, but others stayed at least as well as they were before its use. Addiction to it alone is infrequent and, in comparison to other addictive states, may be relatively benign." A study of eight cases reported in the literature plus one original case led Zondek to the conclusion that: "In view of the fact that it [amphetamine] fulfils most but not all criteria of the World Health Organization's definition for drug addiction, it may be said that the abuse of it lies somewhere between habituation and addiction."

These excerpts from the literature have been chosen to illustrate the degree of controversy that exists with respect to the addictive liabilities of the amphetamines. It is hoped that they also illustrate how the same evidence can lead to almost diametrically opposite judgments and conclusions when an apparently scientific problem involves as well, medical, ethical, social, cultural, and other issues. If this is the case among the experts, the situation must be all the more confusing to the general practitioner and other individuals concerned with the questions of drug abuse. Any non-expert but interested reader, confronted in 1958 with Professor Leake's and Dr. Connell's monographs, would have gathered quite different impressions with respect to the usefulness and merits of the amphetamines on the one hand and to their untoward effects on the other.

CHARACTERISTICS OF DEPENDENCE ON AMPHETAMINES

The great majority of the cases discussed under the heading of psychotic reactions associated with chronic consumption of amphetamines are, of course, instances of prolonged self-administration of the drugs and therefore suitable material to examine with respect to the general characteristics of the dependence. Sixty-two further cases were found in which the chronic abuse did not, at least up to the time of reporting, result in psychotic reactions. They are listed in Table XI. Separate examination is indicated, since it might be argued that those individuals who

TABLE XI

REPORTED CASES OF CHRONIC ABUSE OF AMPHETAMINES WITHOUT DEVELOPMENT OF PSYCHOSIS

Author	Reference	Sex	Age	Drug*	Maximum daily dose	Duration of use	Other drugs taken to excess
Friedenberg (1940) U.S.A.	68	F	30	dl-A SO₄	20 mg	6 mo.	
Hahne (1940) U.S.A.	82	M	49	dl-A SO₄	240 mg	2.5 yr.	alcohol
Cremieux, et al. (1948) France	48	M	32	dl-A SO₄	1500 mg	3 yr.	alcohol
Mitchell & Denton (1950) Canada	128	F	21	d-A SO₄	?	1 yr.	
Gayral & Combes (1950) France	69	F	48	dl-A SO₄; d-A tartrate	50 mg	2 yr.	ether
Knapp (1952) U.S.A.	110	F	30	dl-A SO₄	600 mg	7 yr.	barbiturates
		F	25	dl-A	250 mg	5 yr.	barbiturates
		M	34	dl-A SO₄; d-A SO₄	260 mg	5 yr.	
		M	38	dl-A SO₄; d-A SO₄	200 mg	15 yr.	
		M	48	dl-A SO₄	200 mg	2 yr.	alcohol; narcotics
		M	35	dl-A SO₄	30 mg	4 yr.	
Baruk & Joubert (1953) France	20	F	29	dl-A SO₄	2 tubes	10 yr.	
Atkinson (1954) U.S.A.	15	F	47	d-A SO₄	?	years	thyroid
Bonhoff & Lewrenz (1954) Germany	29	M	30	meth-A HCl	?	6 yr.	alcohol; barbiturates
		M	33	meth-A HCl	?	years	
		M	44	meth-A HCl	30 mg	years	caffeine; barbiturates
		M	36	meth-A HCl	90 mg	2 yr.	barbiturates; narcotics
		M	34	meth-A HCl	6 ampoules	3 yr.	Dolantin; morphine
		M	23	meth-A HCl	4 ampoules	6 mo.	
Corni (1955) Italy	44	M	44	dl-A SO₄; meth-A HCl	50 tablets	?	cocaine; sedatives
		M	47	dl-A SO₄; meth-A HCl	15 tablets	years	morphine
Tolentino & D'Avossa (1957) Italy	176	M	26	dl-A SO₄	10 tablets	7 years	

TABLE XI (concld.)

Author	Reference	Sex	Age	Drug*	Maximum daily dose	Duration of use	Other drugs taken to excess
Zondek (1958) U.K.	202	M	39	d-A SO₄; amytal	200 mg 1300 mg	?	alcohol; barbiturates
Askevold (1959) Norway	14	M	42	amphetamine	?	5 yr.	barbiturates
		M	28	amphetamine	?	2 yr.	alcohol; barbiturates
		M	37	amphetamine	200 mg	3 yr.	barbiturates; morphine
		M	31	amphetamine	?	years	alcohol; barbiturates; morphine
		M	43	amphetamine	500 mg	2 mo.	alcohol
		M	30	amphetamine	?	months	alcohol; morphine
Marley (1960) U.K.	119	M	44	dl-A SO₄	500 mg	10 yr.	alcohol, barbiturates; chloral hydrate
Hay (1962) U.K.	91	F	38	d-A SO₄; amytal	72 mg 460 mg	14 yr.	
McCormick (1962) U.S.A.	127	M	44	d-A SO₄	450 mg	15 yr.	alcohol
Kiloh & Brandon (1962) U.K.	109	F	36	d-A SO₄	200 mg	10 yr.	phenmetrazine
		F	26	dl-A SO₄; amytal	50 mg 320 mg	4 yr.	
McConnell & McIlwaine (1961) U.K. McConnell (1963) U.K.	126 125	25 cases No individual data given					
Oswald & Thacore (1963) U.K.	137	4 cases No individual data given					

*d-A SO₄—d-amphetamine sulfate
dl-A—amphetamine base
dl-A SO₄—amphetamine sulfate
meth-A—methamphetamine base
meth-A HCl—methamphetamine hydrochloride

did develop psychosis abused amphetamines because of latent psychotic traits, and are therefore very unusual cases. Some representative case histories will be described in detail to illustrate the characteristics of the amphetamine type of drug dependence.

Case Histories

CASE 1. In 1940 Hahne (82) reported the case of a 49-year-old man who was a confirmed alcoholic and who requested something to pep him up and to eliminate the craving for alcohol. The author "in the spirit of experimentation" prescribed 20 mg of amphetamine sulfate daily. Some months later the patient reported that amphetamine had completely eliminated the craving for alcohol. He was well and had gained weight. About two years later he reported again because of new regulations requiring prescriptions for amphetamine. He then admitted he was taking about 120 mg daily and sometimes even 240 mg. He stated that he could not carry on without them, since withdrawal produced nervousness, exhaustive fatigue, inability to think straight, and sleeplessness. He had not lost weight and appeared in good health. He had not touched a drop of alcohol since he had begun taking amphetamine.

CASE 2. In 1952 Knapp (110) reported seven original cases of chronic amphetamine abuse, one of which is perhaps the best documented case history of this series. It concerned a 30-year-old nurse who was a captain in the Army Nurse Corps. She had used amphetamine intermittently for seven years and continuously in enormous doses for almost a year while under psychiatric observation. She was the only child of an absentee alcoholic father and a rejecting mother who brought her up under the care of various relatives and a foster home. She went into nursing, about which she had mixed feelings, after her mother remarried. "An impulsive, early marriage ended under unfortunate circumstances. It was followed by a pattern of involvement with older men, usually in a triangular situation, destined to terminate in suffering." She began to rely increasingly on both depressants and amphetamine. After another unhappy relationship she came for psychiatric help. While under observation she continued to have difficult relationships at work and when psychotherapy was interrupted for 3 months she began taking large doses of amphetamine and was hospitalized after taking 600 mg daily for 2 weeks.

"During this period she went through a *phase of activity almost hypomanic in scope*. She worked almost incessantly, lost 60 pounds of weight, and not infrequently went for 72 hours without sleeping. She felt that she was going faster and faster, at a hectic pace. Her need for the drug increased steadily until finally she was stuffing down handfuls, eight or nine 10 mg tablets at a time." Attempts to give up the drug made her terrified of depression and resuming it produced anxiety. Physical examination was essentially negative, except for mild obesity and mild acne. Withdrawal produced some sleepiness and marked irritability and apprehension. Since she demanded large amounts of sedatives it was not possible to tell to what extent the groggy, dazed state that developed was due to withdrawal and how much to the sedatives. After discharge she abstained for 3 months but felt depressed and bitter and at her insistence she was allowed the drug freely once more. She took the drug sporadically often in very large doses for several months but as her therapeutic rapport improved and she concentrated more on her personal problems her need for it diminished. During the last three months of therapy she was taking none.

In summary, her *"relationship to amphetamine"* is described as follows. Objectively the drug made her talkative, cheerful, irritable, and freer than usual to express anger. Subjectively, she experienced euphoria, optimism, energy, and gregariousness which she valued the most. Undesirable effects included initial tachycardia and breathlessness, confused thinking, forgetfulness, rambling talk, persistent tremor, and sores produced by her digging at her arms and face. There was also urinary frequency, dryness of the mouth, and an increase in sexual desire but a decrease in satisfaction. Immediately after stopping the drug her appetite would become ravenous with a "compulsive urge to eat, a desire to fill herself up, or just gobble something down. Both the longing and the hunger would be relieved within 10 minutes by benzedrine." There was also a craving for large amounts of barbiturates and other depressants which she kept more or less in check, often taking both types of drugs together to avoid deep sleep. "Both benzedrine and barbiturates gave her a 'jag' but, she stated, 'there is a big difference'. From the latter she got a confused 'all gone', 'falling apart' feeling, exciting but threatening. Benzedrine left her exhilarated but 'more in control'. At one point her material was formulated in terms of her having two selves, a waking and a dreaming one. She agreed, adding: 'Benzedrine brings out the waking me'."

CASE 3. Bonhoff and Lewrenz (29) reported the case of a 34-year-old medical student who resorted to the use of drugs during a period of great stress including the death of his father, an accident to his daughter, financial troubles, and preparation for his final examinations. At first he took Dolantin and later morphine, but eventually he switched to methamphetamine hydrochloride with which he had become acquainted during the war. He began taking 2 to 3 tablets daily, but increased the dose relatively quickly to 6 ampoules daily. The drug gave him sweats, nausea, dry mouth, palpitations, heart pain, gradually increasing physical weakness, and also a certain increase in libido. His subjective feeling of strength was much greater than his actual endurance. He was unable to concentrate and his notion of time became distorted. He had some sensory illusions but was aware of their nature. His relationship with his wife, from whom he concealed his drug intake, deteriorated. He had to postpone his final examinations, and during a period of depression he attempted to commit suicide. He was able to do without methamphetamine at times by sleeping for a whole weekend or while away on trips with his family, but the threat of his exams led him back to the drug. On admission the patient was anxious, but co-operative and accessible. During the first three days he was dull, apathetic, and sleepy but his former activity returned gradually. On the ninth day he broke off the withdrawal treatment but apparently did not relapse to using drugs. He gave up the study of medicine, took up a job as a salesman, and during subsequent follow-up visits appeared well. He stated that the subjective feelings during withdrawal of morphine or Dolantin, on the one hand, and during withdrawal of methamphetamine on the other were quite different. In the former, one became extremely anguished, excited, and restless, believing one would go half mad with craving, whereas in the latter case one became tired, sleepy, uninterested, physically weak, with an empty feeling inside, unable to concentrate, and without either the strength or the drive to think anything through to the end. He thought it was a rather beneficial state which could be slept off, after which one could return to freshness and strength.

CASE 4. Corni (44) described the case of a 44-year-old man who was admitted to hospital on his own request in order to break his addiction to Stenamina, a mixture of 3 parts methamphetamine hydrochloride and 2 parts amphetamine sulfate. He had a poor family background and a history of addiction to cocaine and of numerous petty crimes. He began using amphetamine when cocaine was difficult to get. At first he mixed it with cocaine but later took it alone, by sniffing, in doses of 15 to 20 tablets per day. At first the drugs produced a sense of well-being, energy, confidence, freedom from worry, and increased sexual power. With time, and despite doses of 40 to 50 tablets daily, these effects wore off and later he felt weakness, vague malaise, and palpitations. Despite medical orders he could not abstain from the drug for more than a week. In hospital the drug was withdrawn over a period of 10 days without incident, but 2 weeks later he was found to be getting tablets from a hidden source and had taken 100 of them. During true withdrawal he suffered from insomnia (he had used sedatives regularly while on amphetamine), irritability, depression, and hostility. At the patient's demand he was allowed to have amphetamine *ad libitum* for 7 days. He became suddenly euphoric, optimistic, active, and talkative and had to take large doses of barbiturates to sleep. He also developed an earthen pallor, tachycardia, tremor, irritability, and precipitate speech. Intensive detoxication therapy was

92

required and even restraint during a period of intense excitement. Physical examination was negative and psychiatric examination indicated a psychopathic personality.

CASE 5. McCormick (127) reported the case of a 44-year-old married man who was a high school teacher and coach, as follows: "Father was alcoholic. Shortly after finishing college he began using alcohol excessively and continued until age 26 when he became a member of Alcoholics Anonymous. Because of a weight problem he began using dexedrine and gradually increased the daily intake to 300 to 450 mg. When he was unable to secure these amounts he became narcoleptic. He developed a severe excoriative dermatitis as well as personality changes and the expense of maintaining this drug caused great hardship to his wife and children. For more than 15 years this man has continued in amphetamine abuse. When unable to secure the drug he has forged prescriptions which led to arrests, court convictions and time served in prison. He has been divorced, re-married and has had sporadic periods of productivity, but he has continued resorting to amphetamines when under any stress or tension."

CASE 6. Kiloh and Brandon (109) reported the following case in 1962: "A 36-year-old woman began to take dexamphetamine as an aid to slimming 10 years ago in amounts of up to 200 mg daily. Even so, there were periods when she remained drowsy and depressed and she failed to lose weight. After four years she stole an E.C. 10 form from her doctor's surgery and wrote out a prescription. This was detected by the pharmacist, who called the police. Her supply of tablets was withdrawn. For four weeks she was confined to bed in a state of collapse, showing marked hypersomnia, and subsequently made a slow return to her normal state. Two years ago she asked her general practitioner for nonhabit forming slimming tablets and was given phenmetrazine. She soon found that she could not manage without these as she felt 'depressed and flat' in spite of a daily intake of 30 tablets. She stole a pad of E.C. 10 forms from a doctor whom she attended as a temporary patient to get an extra supply of tablets, and continued to use it for a year before being caught. During this time she was noted to be restless, overactive, irritable, and unable to settle, doing her housework in spurts. After the withdrawal of her tablets on admission to hospital she became depersonalized, depressed, and sleepy, experienced vivid hypnagogic hallucinations on closing her eyes, and complained that her body felt huge. These features improved after a week, but for a further 10 days or so she felt 'flat' and that she could anticipate people's words and actions, and seemed to know what was going to happen."

With the exception of psychotic breakdowns, these cases are essentially similar to those discussed in the previous chapter, especially with respect to the characteristics of the drug dependence. Periodic or chronic intoxication is present in all of them, as well as a compulsion to continue taking the drug despite various and serious adverse effects. As evidenced in these individual case histories and in the columns indicating the maximum daily doses taken by the patients (Tables VIII and X), tolerance developed in most cases, reaching enormous proportions in some. Psychological dependence on the effects of the drugs is equally evident in all these cases, since the patients were unable to give up the habit on their own and found it most difficult to do so even under supervised conditions. Detrimental effects on the individual have been dramatically and amply demonstrated in the section on amphetamine psychosis, but other serious untoward effects also occur. Frantic, ineffectual, erratic activity, for example, was described in Cases 2, 3, and 6 while under the effect of the drug. During withdrawal the reverse would be true. In Case 3, for example, the patient would sleep for a whole weekend, while in Case 6 abstinence led to a state of prostration lasting several weeks. Irritability, aggressiveness, and loss of judgment are also common features during intoxication.

Although it is difficult to present these effects in a systematic manner, or to properly emphasize their significance in terms of over-all day-to-day conduct, examination of the histories clearly shows that during intoxication these patients show profound alterations of behavior with detrimental effects to themselves and to others. Even though the cases described in this section did not experience psychotic breakdowns, they were disturbed enough to require medical attention and even hospitalization, as illustrated by Cases 2, 3, and 4. The statement of McCormick (127) that "no other group of drugs can affect or change character and personality traits to a greater degree than the amphetamines" seems amply warranted and perhaps not sufficiently emphasized. These alterations of behavior have, of course, a detrimental effect on society, but in addition overt criminal behavior has been described, as in Cases 5 and 6 above. In Case 5 there was hardship to the family of the patient because of the expense of procuring the drug, as well as forgery of prescriptions, arrests, court convictions, and imprisonment.

94

The physical untoward effects, despite the enormous doses taken by these patients, are relatively minor but nevertheless present. There was insomnia requiring large doses of barbiturates in Cases 2 and 4, typical peripheral sympathomimetic symptoms in Cases 2, 3, and 4, and an excoriative dermatitis in Case 5.

Abstinence reactions were generally characterized by sleepiness, depression, lethargy, and similar symptoms, as was very well described by Case 3. This is hardly surprising in the withdrawal of stimulant drugs. Case 2 had a strong craving for food and for barbiturates. In Case 4 there was irritability, hostility, and, paradoxically, insomnia, but that might have been due to the simultaneous withdrawal of barbiturates. The withdrawal reaction was particularly strong and prolonged in Case 6. Craving for the drug during supervised withdrawal in a clinic is well illustrated by Case 4, who managed to consume 100 amphetamine tablets before he was found out. It should be recalled that this patient was voluntarily admitted for the purpose of giving up the use of the drug.

A number of other features of amphetamine abuse are worthy of mention. As the data in Tables VIII and X and the individual case histories show, amphetamine abusers have a high incidence of addiction to or abuse of alcohol and other drugs. Thus, Cases 1 and 5 were confirmed alcoholics prior to their acquaintance with amphetamines. But, interestingly, they were able to do without alcohol while on the latter drugs. In Case 3 amphetamine replaced morphine and in Case 4 cocaine. In Case 2, as well as in many others, there was simultaneous abuse of amphetamines and barbiturates, the latter being taken primarily to counteract the insomnia produced by the former. Case 6 is a typical example of a compulsive eater resorting to amphetamines to reduce, and then becoming strongly dependent on the drug, to the extent of forging prescriptions to secure it. Case 5, at least as judged by this history, is interesting in that the patient did not show any conspicuous signs of abnormal personality prior to the period of extreme stress that led to his first use of drugs.

If the clinical material presented in the previous chapter (Table VIII) and in this section is taken together, and examined in terms of the 1957 definition of addiction by the W.H.O., the following conclusions can be drawn with respect to the addictive properties of the amphetamines. The states of periodic or chronic intoxication produced by the repeated consumption of amphetamines are characterized by: (1) an overpowering desire or need (compulsion) to continue taking the drug and to obtain it by any means; (2) a marked tendency to increase the dose; (3) a psychological dependence on the effects of the drug; and (4) detrimental effects on the individual and on society. Thus, judged clinically, abuse of amphetamines meets all the criteria of addiction with the exception of "generally a physical dependence." Physical dependence is usually judged by the presence of physical symptoms during withdrawal, as is the case in addiction to opiates and alcohol. These are generally absent during withdrawal of amphetamines, but a recent report by Oswald and Thacore (137) strongly suggests that physical alterations in the central nervous system of abusers of amphetamine and amphetamine-like substances do occur.

Oswald and Thacore studied some characteristics of the nocturnal sleep of 6 women who were abusers of amphetamines by recording the electroencephalograms and eye movements during sleep. Three of the women were addicted to Drinamyl (5 mg d-amphetamine sulfate and 32 mg amobarbital per tablet), 2 to phenmetrazine, and one to Durophet (1 part l-amphetamine to 3 parts d-amphetamine).

Recent studies have shown human sleep to consist of two phases referred to as "forebrain" and "hindbrain" phases of sleep. The first is accompanied by high-voltage slow waves and spindles in the EEG, ocular repose, and incomplete relaxation of skeletal muscle. Hindbrain sleep is accompanied by bursts of conjugate rapid eye movements and an EEG of fairly low voltage with periods of characteristic saw-toothed waves of 2–3 cps. It appears after a period of forebrain sleep of about 70 minutes and recurs cyclically, occupying 4–6 discrete periods of the night. It occupies about 10 minutes of the first 2 hours of sleep and about 22 per cent of the whole night's rest.

During withdrawal in these patients, the hindbrain sleep began as soon as 4 minutes (normal about 70 minutes) after onset of sleep and occupied up to 70 minutes (normal about 10 minutes)

96

in the first 2 hours and up to 48 per cent (normal about 22 per cent) of the whole night. Return to normal took 3 to 8 weeks. If the drugs were restored the return of the sleep pattern to normal was immediate, that is, during drug intake the sleep was essentially normal. The authors concluded that the patients were physically dependent on the drugs, since dependence means that some physiological function is normal in the addict, becomes abnormal on withdrawal, and returns to normal if the drug is given again. Since barbiturates were consumed simultaneously with amphetamines by only 3 of the 6 patients, while the disturbances were shown by all 6, these effects are presumably due to withdrawal of the amphetamines and related drugs, although the authors do not discuss this point. The significance of these findings goes beyond the field of the amphetamines. In the authors' own words: "We believe this to be the first demonstration of an abnormality both easily measurable and long-persisting (one to two months) in any kind of human abstinence syndrome."

In 1964 Wilson and Beacon (199) published some interesting results of an investigation into the habituating properties of an amphetamine-barbiturate mixture. An experiment was designed to find out the extent to which patients were habituated to Drinamyl which they were receiving from their doctors for therapeutic purposes. Habituation was stated here to mean a condition involving psychic dependence resulting from the repeated consumption of the drugs. The investigation was carried out in Liverpool with the co-operation of 14 general practitioners and 58 patients, 47 of whom were women.

Under what was intended to be double-blind conditions, the patients were to receive Drinamyl (triangular blue tablets containing 5 mg of d-amphetamine and 32 mg of amobarbital) for four 2-week periods, round white tablets with the same amounts of amphetamine and barbiturate for one 2-week period, and triangular blue tablets containing only lactose for two 2-week periods. At the end of each period the patients answered a questionnaire designed to establish their reaction to the tablets. In fact many patients defected from the trial after the fourth period. The results deal only with the first 4 periods which in 19 cases included all 3 preparations, in another 19 included Drinamyl and dummy Drinamyl, and in 15 cases true Drinamyl only. At the end of each period the patients were asked whether or not they could do without the tablets. Twenty-two of the 53 patients who finished 4 periods said that they could do without, while 31 said they could not. In fact, however, only 7 of the first group actually agreed to stop when asked to do so. Therefore it would appear that 46 of the 53 were really dependent upon pill-taking. Of these 46 patients, 23 were unable to distinguish placebo tablets from true Drinamyl; these were classed as "psychologically dependent" by the authors. The other 23 either recognized the placebos, or were so heavily dependent upon the drugs that the authors did not consider it advisable to give them placebos; these were all classified as "pharmacologically dependent." Of the 19 who received the same drugs in the form of a round white tablet, 8 considered it equally effective, while 11 found it different. Yet, oddly enough, almost the same proportion of each group were among those classed as psychologically dependent (7/8 of the first group and 8/11 of the second).

The authors concluded that the "psychologically dependent" patients, that is those who found the placebo acceptable, should not be given the active drugs. In contrast, patients who were able to distinguish between the true drugs and the placebo might, in the authors' opinion, be given the drugs justifiably if adequate psychiatric help is unavailable and if the drugs are given "under carefully controlled conditions." The authors state that, in the latter group, Drinamyl satisfies all the characteristics laid down for drugs of habituation, but presumably not of addiction because, "signs or symptoms of a true withdrawal syndrome were not detected."

A minor criticism is that the term double-blind is not really applicable to this study, since the patients were deliberately being asked to compare two physical formulations of the same drugs. A more important objection is the authors' use of the terms "psychological" and "pharmacological" dependence. It is implied that pharmacological dependence is physical rather than psychological. This is a confusing use of the terms because there can be psychological dependence on the pure pharmacological effects of the drug, even in the absence of physical dependence as shown by the lack of a withdrawal reaction. Despite these comments, the study clearly showed that a high proportion of patients receiving the drug were highly dependent on it, in one way or another, and that some had developed a considerable degree of tolerance. The authors refer to one patient who took 15 tablets daily and would have taken more, except that it spoiled her appetite. They state further that "a few patients take as many as 50 tablets per day." Moreover, though they consider the use of Drinamyl justifiable in certain cases "under carefully controlled conditions," their own evidence indicates that these conditions may be very difficult to achieve. They found for example, that patients often kept stores of tablets at home, did not return them on request, took the whole 2-week supply in 2 or 3 days, and stole or forged prescriptions during the investigation, and one patient even stole 420 tablets from the office of a participating physician.

It must be pointed out that Drinamyl is a mixture of amphetamine and a barbiturate, and that the contribution of the latter to the over-all effects cannot be ignored. However, from the descriptions of the subjective effects given by the patients in this study it would appear that the amphetamine action is the predominant one, at least with respect to the patients' desire to continue using the drug.

The findings of Oswald and Thacore and of Wilson and Beacon indicate that both physical and psychological dependence can develop upon prolonged use of amphetamines. Although the physical dependence suggested by this evidence is not severe it appears none the less to be present.

It should be evident from this discussion that addiction (as formerly defined by the W.H.O. Expert Committee) to amphetamines does exist, and that when it does it constitutes a serious problem, at least from the point of view of the individual concerned. It should be equally evident that abuse of these stimulants ranges from occasional use for some specific purpose, through various degrees of habituation to addiction, much as happens with alcohol or barbiturates. Indeed, in the light of the evidence reviewed here, the new W.H.O. definition of "drug

99

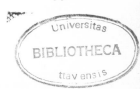

dependence of amphetamine type" (p. 79) does not appear to give sufficient emphasis to the severity of the dependence which can develop.

Two further points concerning the question of "addiction" to amphetamines deserve comment. One is that in much of the pertinent literature the prototype of addiction is tacitly or explicitly considered to be that produced by the opiates and the inevitable comparisons follow. If a drug produces a picture essentially similar to that of the consumption of the opiates, particularly a "characteristic" withdrawal syndrome, then it is easily defined as addictive. If it does not, its addictive liabilities are questioned. This tendency to *compare* has perhaps interfered with the objective examination of the characteristics of amphetamine dependence. For example, it has often been stated that withdrawal of amphetamines does not produce "characteristic" abstinence symptoms, and yet in the vast majority of cases, sleepiness, lethargy, and depression are described as present and marked. Why should abnormally prolonged sleep or lethargy not be considered as "characteristic" symptoms of the withdrawal of a stimulant drug? This almost suggests that in this context the term "characteristic" is used to mean similar to the withdrawal symptoms seen in other addictions, rather than typical of the withdrawal of the drug in question. If depressant drugs such as morphine and alcohol give rise to withdrawal syndromes characterized by marked degrees of excitability it is difficult to understand why depression and sleepiness should not be considered characteristic symptoms of the withdrawal of a stimulant drug.

The second point refers to what might be termed internal as opposed to external withdrawal. When the rate of degradation and excretion of a drug is high, as is the case with morphine (58a), suspension of intake and disappearance of the drug from the internal environment are separated by an interval of only a few hours, after which the individual can be considered to be in a true state of withdrawal. When, on the other hand, the rate of excretion is low, as with the amphetamines (42), the interval between suspension of intake and disappearance of the drug from the internal environment is prolonged. During this time (days) the individual is undergoing gradual rather than abrupt withdrawal.

This situation is somewhat comparable to the one that obtains during the gradual external withdrawal of drugs with a high rate of elimination. It is noteworthy that even among the opiates the rate of elimination is correlated with the severity of the withdrawal symptoms. Methadone, for example, is eliminated much more slowly than morphine (189a) and its withdrawal symptoms are much milder (98b). Thus the absence of marked abstinence symptoms after chronic abuse of amphetamines may well be due to the slow rather than abrupt internal withdrawal.

Therefore neither the dissimilarity between the withdrawal symptoms of morphine and those of amphetamines, nor the relative mildness of the latter, can be used as arguments for the concept that the amphetamines are non-addictive.

Since many case histories indicate that the patients began to use amphetamines in place of other addictive drugs which they could no longer obtain, it has been argued that the amphetamines are mere substitutes rather than primary drugs of addiction. The specious implication here is that abuse of a substitute is *per se* a less serious problem than abuse of the original drug. However, it could equally be argued that the opiates are in many instances mere substitutes for marihuana, alcohol, or amphetamines. Substitution of one drug for another has often more to do with opportunity and availability than with the specific pharmacological properties of the drug. What this evidence does indicate, however, is that many individuals are quite unable to function without the intake of drugs and will resort to one or another in a trial and error fashion, the end result depending on their make-up, on the one hand, and on the effects and pharmacological properties of the drug on the other. Addiction cannot occur without the interaction between a drug with certain characteristics and a receptor organism, also possessing certain characteristics.

A related question, even more important from a social or public health point of view, is the extent of this type of drug abuse. As early as 1950, Keyserlingk (108b) reported that of 100 patients admitted to his hospital because of drug addiction, 13 were abusers of methamphetamine and the majority of these developed a toxic psychosis. He also referred to an earlier statement by Nau that 16 of 66 drug addicts, admitted during a 6-month period to the Berlin Medico-Legal Institute, were abusers of methamphetamine. The literature shows that amphetamine addiction constituted an extremely serious problem in Japan after the second world war and a rising problem in Great Britain in recent years. Because of the sharpness with which the social and medical aspects of the problem have been focussed, the evidence is given in some detail below.

THE PROBLEM OF AMPHETAMINE ABUSE IN JAPAN

Reports of widespread amphetamine abuse in Japan have been made by Noda (133), Hara, *et al.* (86), Kaga (106), Masaki (121), Sano and Nagasaka (157), and Tatetsu (173), among others.

Amphetamines, which had been used by the Japanese armed forces during the second world war, were apparently dumped at the end of the war and a flourishing black market arose. According to Masaki abuse of these drugs was first noticed in 1945 and increased markedly after 1948. The drugs most commonly used were amphetamine sulfate and methamphetamine hydrochloride, referred to generally as Philopon and the abuse as philoponism. Information provided by the Ministry of Welfare in May, 1954, showed that 10,148 persons had been taken into custody because of offences against the Awakening Drug [Amphetamines] Control Law and that 52 per cent of these were addicts. One estimate of the number of abusers in Japan in 1954 was 500,000–600,000, of which 50 per cent were considered addicts. The estimate of the Japan Pharmacist Association was 1.5 million.

Noda (133) made a study of 136 addicts from Kurume, where 1,000 out of a population of 90,000, or 1.1 per cent, were amphetamine addicts. Since most of the addicts were men between the ages of 16 and 25 years they amounted to 5 per cent of the younger generation. Noda also reported that 4 per cent of 500 students in one high school and 2 per cent of 2,000 workers in one factory were addicts. Hara, *et al.* (86), studied amphetamine poisoning in 52 cases at the Numazu Mental Hospital. Kaga (106) reported a statistical study of 117 addicts admitted to the Musashino Mental Hospital between 1949 and 1954. The study of Sano and Nagasaka (157) concerned 599 cases of methamphetamine abuse in Osaka seen by the authors between 1949 and 1953, and Tatetsu (173) reported on 492 cases of methamphetamine psychosis.

All the reports agree that the highest incidence of amphetamine abuse occurred in young men from a low socio-economic class. For example, Noda stated that his group ranged in age from 16 to 27 years, but that 70 per cent were between 18 and 23. Twenty-six per cent of these were unemployed with a long history of addiction. More than half had begun to use the drug in their teens, and the length of the addiction ranged from 6 months (29 per cent) to 4 years (4 per cent). According to Kaga (106), 80 per cent of his cases were below 30 years of age and 70 per cent had started taking amphetamines before they were 25. Seventy-two per cent of the largest series, reported by Sano and Nagasaka (157), were between 20 and 29 years of age; 90 per cent were men, 62 per cent were single, and 45 per cent were unemployed. Masaki also states that a survey carried out in 1954 showed that 33 per cent of juveniles confined to reformatories were familiar with amphetamines, indicating a close relation between juvenile delinquency and amphetamine abuse.

Important contributory factors to this widespread abuse of amphetamines were, according to Masaki, the availability of a large military stock of the drugs after the surrender of Japan and the spiritual collapse that followed the defeat. But by 1955 it was apparent that solicitation by illegal distributors had become an important factor. Of 116 addicts admitted to hospitals because of mental impairment by amphetamines, the motives for the abuse were: night amusement, 43 cases; solicitation, 31; curiosity, 24; deception, 8; to improve performance, 8; desperation, 2; studying, 1; and obesity, 1. According to this study the psychological make-up of these patients included "weak-mindedness" in 61 cases, emotional instability in 25, lack of self-confidence in 16, conceit in 5, and explosive temper in 1. Noda also states that most of his patients were "weak-minded" individuals with a sociable, jovial, showy, inconstant, selfish personality.

The most common mode of administration was by intravenous

injection. According to Noda most patients begin with doses of 1 to 3 ampoules (3–9 mg) per day, but rapidly increase it to a maximum of 200 ampoules per day. Sixty-five per cent of his series used 1 to 10 ampoules daily. In general, the longer standing the addiction the higher the dose, but most patients had reached their maximum dose within 4 months. Hara, *et al.* (86), state that the daily dosage ranged from 10 to 160 ml. The exact concentration was not known because most products were manufactured illegally, but from the results of animal experiments it was estimated at 2 to 3 mg per ml. Masaki stated that a survey in 1951–52 indicated that 6 per cent of the illegal products did not contain amphetamines at all.

Noda stated that the effects of the first injection of amphetamine in most patients were mental stimulation, decrease in need for sleep, and increase in activity, although 9 patients felt no effect at all and 6 had headaches and discomfort. The principal symptoms, and the number of instances of each, in 75 patients who were observed more thoroughly are shown in Table XII. Noda

TABLE XII

FREQUENCY OF SYMPTOMS OF AMPHETAMINE TOXICITY AS DESCRIBED BY NODA (133)

Somatic		Mental	
Thirst	75	Irritability	71
Anorexia	72	Anxiety	68
Emaciation	70	Inactivity	64
Polyuria	68	Loss of memory	62
Paleness	68	Delusions	39
Decreased libido	61	Hallucinations	30
Palpitations	59	Logorrhea	18
Dizziness	50		
Perspiration	48		

stated that long-term addicts looked like "living skeletons." The auditory and visual hallucinations and the ideas of persecution and of reference were not accompanied by disturbances of consciousness and the picture resembled cocaine intoxication. Of 28 alcoholics in the group, 15 had ceased to drink and 3 did not get drunk despite heavy drinking.

Hara, *et al.* (86), described the major physical symptoms as anorexia, insomnia, thirst, perspiration, and palpitations, and the major mental symptoms as ideas of reference, talkativeness, hyperactivity, auditory hallucinations, and automatism. According to Kaga (106) the principal symptoms were hallucinations and delusions. Disturbances of consciousness were rare and the picture resembled schizophrenia except that it cleared up within 15–30 days in most cases.

Sano and Nagasaka (157) found that 21.9 per cent of their 599 cases suffered from addiction without psychosis, 62.1 per cent had addiction with psychosis which cleared promptly on withdrawal, and in 10 per cent the psychosis had become chronic. Generally the symptoms resembled those of schizophrenia rather than those of other toxic psychoses. There was no disturbance of consciousness. Either slowing or intense pressure of thought, imaginary experiences, absentmindedness, and delusions predominated, especially paranoidal ideas. More than 50 per cent had auditory hallucinations and somatic hallucinations were frequent. Disturbances of volition included hypokinesia and stupor in 45 per cent, abulia in 68 per cent and restlessness and hyperkinesia in 38 per cent. Disturbances of mood were: manic, 24 per cent; depressive, 15 per cent; apathetic, 57 per cent; irritable, 51 per cent; anxious, 43 per cent. Disturbances of thought and sensation were: absentmindedness, 24 per cent; and sensory disturbances, especially auditory hallucinations, 68 per cent. Psychiatrically the pictures were classified as: schizophrenic-like, 45 per cent; manic depressive, 5 per cent; mixed manic or depressive moods together with schizophrenic symptoms, 40 per cent; and organic forms, 10 per cent. Despite the high proportion of schizophrenic-like symptoms, communication was good and automatism was never seen. The 10 per cent who did not recover after withdrawal were classified as schizophrenia provoked by amphetamines.

Tatetsu (173), who studied 492 cases of methamphetamine psychosis, classified the mental disturbances observed into two major groups. Eight per cent of the cases were referred to as psychopathic-like and included one subgroup described as vulgar, threatening, and irritable, and another described as weak, hypotonic, strengthless, and effeminate. Ninety-two per cent of the cases were described as psychotic-like, including schizophrenoids (19 per cent), manic depressive (23 per cent), mixed schizophrenoid and manic depressive (19 per cent), and apathetic exhausted states (31 per cent). In Tatetsu's view, the schizophrenoids differ from true schizophrenics in that they always maintained contact with reality despite such gross disturbances as hallucinations and catatonia, and that the incidence of true schizophrenia in their siblings and parents is only one-third as high as in the families of schizophrenics, although considerably higher than in the general population. Bielschowsky stains of brain tissue sections of schizophrenoids do not show the axone cylinder changes which Tatetsu thinks are typical of true schizophrenia. The manic-depressive pictures were similar to endogenous psychoses, but the manic states predominated. The apathetic-exhausted states lasted about a month in most cases and were then replaced by psychopathic or psychotic states of milder degree. In general the psychopathic-like cases had used smaller doses than the psychotic-like cases and for shorter periods, but among the latter there was no clear-cut relation between the dose and the severity of the psychosis.

Most of these authors agree that withdrawal led to rapid recovery in the majority of the patients with psychotic symptoms, and was undramatic in the others, being accompanied characteristically by sleepiness, fatigue, and apathy. Other than prompt withdrawal of the drug, the treatment used by these authors was symptomatic, including electroshock therapy in patients who became extremely irritable and emotional (Noda), intravenous injection of apomorphine after several electroshock treatments, or continuous administration of chlorpromazine or a mixture of chlorpromazine and reserpine (Masaki).

The prognosis was generally considered bad. Noda reported that of 75 patients who had stopped taking amphetamines by themselves, only 2 were still off the drug at the time of writing. The others were able to abstain for from 10 days to 3 months, and 23 had tried without success. He also stated that 6 patients became narcotic addicts while 3 narcotic addicts became addicted to amphetamines. Tatetsu stated that, although a significant proportion of methamphetamine addicts (42 per cent in one series) were able to stop by themselves, the relapse rate was high. In this series, complete remission of the toxic symptoms occurred in 36 per cent of the patients. Thirty-seven per cent were able to go home but unable to work, one committed suicide, and 26 per cent were obliged to remain in hospital.

According to Noda 61 per cent of the patients had been involved in antisocial behavior, and Masaki stated that crimes were committed by these patients to obtain amphetamines and also as a result of the effects of the drug on their behavior. He says that 31 out of 60 convicted murderers in Japan during May and June, 1954, had some connection with misuse of amphetamines.

This situation led the Japanese government to enact severe legislation against the indiscriminate use of amphetamines. In 1949 the use of these drugs was restricted to cases under medical care. In 1951 the Awakening Drug Control Law was enacted, by which importation of amphetamines into Japan was prohibited, and possession, manufacture, sale, and purchase of the drugs were severely restricted. The law was made even stricter in 1954 and again in 1955. At the same time the government set up the Awakening Drug Countermeasure Headquarters under the Minister of Welfare, to instruct the public on the problem and to gain their co-operation in eliminating it.

THE CURRENT PROBLEM OF AMPHETAMINE ABUSE IN THE UNITED KINGDOM

During the last few years, several reports and numerous editorials (6–11) and letters to the editor have appeared in the British medical literature, testifying to the widespread abuse of amphetamines, barbiturates, combinations of the two, and also of the newer anorectics such as phenmetrazine and diethylpropion. Some of these reports which deserve special consideration are summarized below.

Struck by the fact that an appreciable number of patients in Newcastle-upon-Tyne were taking large quantities of amphetamines and amphetamine-like substances, Kiloh and Brandon

(109) made a study of the amounts of these drugs prescribed in the city, of the methods used by the patients to obtain their supplies, and of the incidence of habituation and addiction in the population. Their clinical experience had already indicated that amphetamine consumption played a significant role in the "genesis and symptomatology of the psychiatric disturbances demanding admission." Their male patients were mainly psychopaths who developed amphetamine psychosis. In contrast, the women were primarily neurotic, inadequate, and prone to depression, and amphetamines tended to aggravate their condition.

A survey of National Health Service prescriptions dispensed in Newcastle during May and November, 1960, revealed that 4,052 or 3.4 per cent of the total issued during May, and 3,077 (2.5 per cent) of those issued during November were for some form of amphetamine preparation. These prescriptions and those issued in two city hospitals were equivalent to a total monthly prescription of 200,000 5-mg tablets, of which 53 per cent were dispensed as Drinamyl (d-amphetamine sulfate and amobarbital). Since the population of Newcastle-upon-Tyne was 269,389 at that time, the amount of amphetamines prescribed would be roughly 45 mg, or nine 5-mg tablets per year for every man, woman, and child. The authors note that these are minimum figures, as they do not take into account private prescriptions, amphetamines sold without prescription, and supplies obtained elsewhere.

There was no evidence of organized illicit traffic in amphetamines but there were indications of small-scale peddlers who obtained the drugs from their own doctors, using one subterfuge or another, and then sold the drugs at a profit. Most patients, however, obtained the drugs directly from their doctors, and when this was not enough they requested prescriptions from all the doctors in a group practice, claimed repeatedly that either the prescription or the tablets had been lost, obtained prescriptions for various members of the family, registered with a number of different doctors using false names if necessary, altered prescriptions and, finally, stole blank E.C. 10 forms and forged the prescriptions. Although no cases of forged prescriptions had been reported to the police between July, 1959, and June, 1960, 22 cases, mostly women, were reported between July, 1960, and December, 1961.

The authors concluded that the responsibility for this state of affairs lies partly with the patients and the pharmacists, but primarily with the doctors. The retail pharmacists were considered responsible to the extent that they sometimes provide these drugs without prescription, that they repeatedly re-fill private prescriptions, or that they do not do enough to call attention to the abuse of the drugs. The doctors were held even more responsible because they prescribe these drugs too readily and uncritically, often under strong pressure from the patients themselves.

This study was extended by a co-operative investigation carried out by general practitioners in the Newcastle area, reported separately by Brandon and Smith (31). The investigation indicated that one per cent of all registered patients, or an estimated 2600 patients in Newcastle-upon-Tyne, were receiving amphetamines. Since about 200,000 tablets were prescribed each month, these patients were receiving about 77 tablets each per month. Eighty-five per cent of the patients were women, usually housewives between 36 and 45 years of age. It was estimated that more than 20 per cent of them were habituated or addicted, "having received the drug for prolonged periods, showing dependence upon it, and proving resistant to withdrawal." The most common reasons for taking the drugs were depression, fatigue, obesity, and anxiety.

Kiloh and Brandon concluded: "The abuse of amphetamines in Newcastle-upon-Tyne is a problem of appreciable size and one that is growing. For the most part it is covert and there seems to be little general appreciation of its existence. There is no reason to suppose that Newcastle-upon-Tyne is unique in this matter, and it is likely that the problem is a national and not merely a local one."

Under the title of "Amphetamine Substances and Mental Illness in Northern Ireland," McConnell and McIlwaine (126) and McConnell (125) reported on 31 cases of amphetamine abuse accompanied by mental and other symptoms seen during a three-year period at the Department of Mental Health of Queen's

University in Belfast. This amounted to about 2 per cent of the total number of referrals, but since the presenting symptoms are not specific and urinary tests for amphetamines are not routine it was considered that the incidence of these conditions was probably higher. Six of these cases presented with psychotic symptoms, 20 were considered to be dependent on the drugs, and 5 suffered from miscellaneous symptoms attributable to amphetamines. They have already been discussed under the appropriate headings. The authors considered this as strong evidence of misuse of amphetamines in Northern Ireland and remarked that: "These substances have few and very limited therapeutic indications and their widespread use greatly exceeds any possible need."

Oswald and Thacore (137), in the article already discussed, state that addiction to amphetamines is common in Edinburgh. They are also of the opinion that the "therapeutic indications for amphetamines are to-day becoming vanishingly slight" and that "these drugs, and drugs with comparable actions, such as diethylpropion, are dangerous drugs in fact if not yet in law."

In a recent publication, Connell (43) discussed several aspects of the problem of amphetamine misuse in Great Britain. His general views on the controversial question of addiction have already been discussed. In addition, he presented further evidence of amphetamine abuse. This included reference to 10 cases "who could be considered as amphetamine addicts, if the 1950 W.H.O. definition is used." They were seen while gathering material for his study of amphetamine psychosis, but did not develop psychotic symptoms. After presenting 8 capsule histories to illustrate the extremes to which these patients will go to obtain their drugs, he concluded: "The full stories of these patients are pathetic in the extreme and the amount of family disruption, marital disharmony, and harm to the children I have seen, due to the effects of amphetamine misuse, is widespread."

Connell also described two case histories to illustrate the problem of abuse of Drinamyl or "purple hearts" among teenagers in Britain. One was a boy of 15 who was introduced to Drinamyl by a friend in a West London cafe. He also tried amyl nitrite ("it's not very good"), Benzedrine ("not all that good"), Dexedrine

("all right"), and marihuana ("not so good as purple hearts").
Drinamyl made him "feel good" and enabled him to talk, but
"when they start wearing off you feel miserable and as though
you want some more to feel better." On one occasion when he
took 50 tablets, 5 at a time every 5 or 10 minutes, he developed
psychotic symptoms referred to as the "horrors." He took the
drug during weekends in the West End but not during the week.
The other boy, aged 17, began taking Drinamyl when he was 15
years and 3 months old and eventually reached a dose of 70
tablets per day. He had had several attacks of the "horrors," had
had to sell or pawn most of his possessions to obtain money for
the drugs, and was now unable to keep his jobs because he was
too sleepy during week days. He also took the drug during weekends in West End "clubs." Marihuana had no effect and he
refrained from heroin because it was too dangerous.

Connell suggested that the teenage "purple heart" problem
may differ from adult habituation and addiction in several respects. Teenage abuse of these drugs involves a cultural factor in
that it is an acceptable group activity. The compulsive element is
less apparent since the drugs are taken during weekends only.
And finally "the teenagers who take these drugs seem to contain
a high proportion of emotionally immature, passive individuals
who, during adolescence, have a great need to show spirit, inde-
pendence, positivity of behavior—the more aggressive features of
behavior." Since many adolescents with similar problems eventually achieve emotional maturity, Connell does not consider that
these individuals will inevitably "develop into chronic personality
disorders, including the disorder of drug addiction." In his
opinion, however, a certain proportion of them will become drug
addicts, much as others who drink heavily at this age will become
alcoholics. This outcome is further favored by the cultural setting
which involves contact with adult sexual perverts, addicts to
opiates, and cocaine and marihuana users. He feels that, in contrast with the problem of alcoholism, stringent measures to control
the availability of this type of drugs "may in fact protect the
teenage population provided that they are used early enough and
before the total culture of the community comes to regard drug
taking as being normal, acceptable and even desirable."

Despite the occurrence of serious abuse of amphetamines by some members of the adult population, many individuals with mild emotional disorders do profit from the use of these drugs in moderate doses, even if taken for prolonged periods of time. Because of this and other considerations, Connell does not favor the complete withdrawal of amphetamines from circulation that has been proposed by certain authors. He suggests, instead, the following measures to prevent the most serious dangers.

1. Close supervision of drug-taking by medical practitioners. This could be reinforced by referring to the amphetamines as drugs of addiction so that they will be taken seriously, by education of the medical profession in the risks involved, and by placing the drugs in a much stricter category of control.

2. Criminal prosecution for possession of the drugs except when they have been obtained under medical prescription.

3. Close supervision of imports of the drug.

4. Marketing of the drugs in less attractive ways.

5. Careful selection of patients for amphetamine therapy, positive rather than negative prescribing, and regular evaluation for continuous therapy.

6. Prophylactic measures such as child care and psychiatry to prevent the emotional disorders of later life which underlie amphetamine misuse.

There has been a steady stream of letters to the editor in the British medical literature, referring to the increasing problem of amphetamine abuse in recent years. A number of important points recur throughout this correspondence. Several letters (66, 123, 147, and 34) have called attention to the frequency with which obese women, originally using amphetamines for weight reduction, become psychically dependent or addicted to the drugs. This dependence or addiction is revealed by the development of tolerance (34) and by an inability to stop taking the drugs. Some of the correspondents have referred to the extremes to which patients will go to obtain supplies, ranging from constant pressure upon the physician to theft and forgery of prescriptions (147 and 198). This type of amphetamine abuse, initiated through physician's prescriptions, would appear to be quite widespread (66, 123, 147, 178, 124, 34, and 139). There is apparently no organized illicit traffic in amphetamines so far (184), but this may be because, in the opinion of some of the writers (123, 72, 139, and 30), many physicians do not take seriously enough the risks of taking these drugs and give repeat prescriptions without enough critical judgment. McConnell (124) reported that the General Health Services Board for Northern Ireland took steps in 1961 "to acquaint all general practitioners of the problem, and there has been a subsequent reduction in the number of patients seen whose symptoms were attributable to amphetamine preparations."

A different type of problem is presented by the widespread use of amphetamines by teenagers who take them without medical indication in the course of their social activities. Case reports by Connell have already been presented and a similar case was described by Bachrich (17).

According to an editorial in *Lancet* (12) Scott and Willcox of the Maudsley Hospital examined the urines of 558 adolescents (mostly boys between 12 and 17 years of age) admitted to London remand homes and found amphetamine-like substances in 18 per cent of them. Physical and psychiatric examination had revealed only a fifth this number of amphetamine takers. The boys also minimized the risks of addiction and psychoses despite evidence to the contrary. Supplies of amphetamines and amphetamine-barbiturate combinations were obtained from pushers. The boys were introduced to the drugs in "clubs" and some even in schools but rarely by a doctor. The reasons for indulgence—self-consciousness and social mimicry, for example—were similar to those of alcoholics, but the teenagers preferred Coca-Cola to alcohol. The majority of the boys took the drugs only during weekends, but a small minority with severe personality disorders did so all the time, increased the dosage, and often progressed to cocaine or opiate addiction. A comparison between 50 amphetamine takers and a control group of delinquents failed to show any definite relation between amphetamine abuse and type or severity of antisocial behavior.

According to Scott (162) it seems likely, although unproven until the incidence of amphetamine-taking in the general teenage population is known, that "adolescent drug-taking may prove to have similar roots in opportunity and predisposition as delinquency, and that, like delinquency, it has a large 'fringe' component and a small 'hard core'."

The only discordant view encountered in this survey was that of Stungo (172) who stated: "There is ample proof that so-called addiction and habituation to amphetamines occur predominantly in those addicted to other drugs and in neurotic subjects who crave medication. A study of the past history of an 'addict' to amphetamine invariably reveals unequivocal evidence of psychopathy, and I consider the 'addiction' generally to be merely another manifestation of instability, maladjustment, or psychotic behavior, rather than a disease *per se.*"

AMPHETAMINE ABUSE IN THE UNITED STATES
AND CANADA

In contrast to the evidence of a serious and growing problem of amphetamine and barbiturate abuse in Great Britain, the current American literature on this subject is scanty and rather confusing.

The official position of the Council on Drugs of the American Medical Association in 1963 (45) was that the abuse of amphetamines is rare when they are prescribed by physicians. The Council recognized that "under appropriate circumstances, widespread abuse of these stimulants may occur" as, for example in postwar Japan, but it added: "In the U.S. at this time compulsive abuse of the amphetamines (or of barbiturates) constitutes such a small problem that additional measures to control such abuse seem unnecessary." The Council felt that further legislation of the type that now applies to the narcotics is neither necessary nor desirable because it would create greater problems by shifting the responsibility for control from physicians to law enforcement agencies. The scarcity of recent reports of amphetamine abuse by American authors would appear to be in agreement with the statement of the Council. However, the few reports available, such as those of Hampton (85), Rickman *et al.* (150), McCormick (127), and Breitner (31a) describing rather large series of psychotic

114

reactions associated with amphetamine abuse, would suggest that the problem may be bigger than is generally appreciated.

Further evidence in this respect was presented recently by Schremly and Solomon (160). These authors made a study of the incidence of drug abuse and drug addiction among all the patients admitted to the Emergency Floor of the Boston City Hospital between October, 1961, and May, 1962. This was done with the co-operation of the house officers who were asked to diagnose and report to the authors each new case. In addition the authors themselves interviewed every twentieth admission during a 24-hour period at weekly intervals from December, 1960, to March, 1962. During the 8-month period approximately 100,000 patients were admitted, and among them 82 cases of drug abuse or addiction were found. This was in contrast with the 10 cases reported to either the Boston City Hospital or the Commonwealth of Massachusetts Food and Drug Division. Of the 82 cases, 40 were addicted to various opiates, 4 to both heroin and barbiturates, 17 to barbiturates, 7 to various tranquilizers, 6 to amphetamines, 3 to amphetamines and barbiturates, and 5 to other sedatives and analgesics. The house officers detected 28 cases during the 4 months they worked alone and 41 cases while working with the authors. The authors detected another 13 cases.

The findings indicated a large discrepancy between the number of drug abusers and addicts detected and the number reported to official agencies (only 7 per cent). The authors concluded that "there may be far more drug abusers and addicts in the general population than has ever been suspected (apparently 3 per 1000)" and that the official statistics may underestimate the true incidence of drug abuse and addiction by 2 orders of magnitude, both because of a failure to report diagnosed cases and because of a lack of interest and attention to the problem of diagnosis. It should be emphasized that about 10 per cent of all cases of drug abuse involved amphetamines.

This work, and the surveys carried out in Great Britain, strongly indicate that estimates of incidence of amphetamine abuse based on general impressions or on reported cases can be totally misleading. Evidence of a different nature, stemming from the lay press, government agencies, and congress, also suggests that abuse of psychotropic drugs generally and amphetamines in particular is widespread in the United States.

In 1960 A. S. Fleming (64), then Secretary of Health, Education and Welfare, reported that a survey, initially concentrated on the bootlegging of amphetamines to truck drivers revealed extensive illicit traffic of these drugs in the United States. It was found that more than 200 operators of truck stops were selling tablets and more than 800,000 tablets were found in the hands of wholesale peddlers. One had 625,000 tablets in his house. Since the production of amphetamines in the United States in 1958 was about 75,000 pounds, or 3.5 billion tablets, or about 20 tablets for every man, woman, and child, the Secretary felt that bootlegging must be more widespread than had so far been found. He also stated that the drug had been found on drivers in a number of fatal highway accidents, and that there was other circumstancial evidence to implicate the drug in these accidents. Under the federal Food, Drug and Cosmetic Act it is illegal to dispense these drugs without a doctor's prescription but the Secretary did not consider that law adequate to cope with the problem and proposed several ways of improving the enforcement program.

According to Walsh (187), in August, 1964, Food and Drug Commissioner G. P. Larrick, testifying at the Senate hearings dealing with the Dodd bill on psychotropic drugs, stated that truck stops have become major centres of distribution for the black market in amphetamines, and also in barbiturates, which the truck drivers take to counteract the lingering effects of the former drugs. In 1964, Food and Drug Act inspectors had spent approximately 56 inspector man years (out of a total of 687) investigating illegal drug sales and were facing increasingly hazardous conditions in their work. According to Larrick amphetamines, purchased from the manufacturers at $1 per thousand, are sold wholesale in the black market at $30 to $40 per thousand and retail at $50 to $100. He also stated that at least enough drugs had been produced in 1962 to make over 9 billion doses of barbiturates and amphetamines and that probably half of these found their way to the black market. These figures were considered incomplete because of inadequate records kept by several manufacturers and because two of the largest pharmaceutical firms declined to provide information.

Senator Dodd stated at the hearings (187) that an investigation carried out by his subcommittee on the use of non-narcotic drugs by young people had led to the following conclusions:

The illegal use of these drugs is increasing at a fantastic rate among juveniles and young adults.

The use of these drugs has a direct causal relationship to increased crimes of violence.

The use of these drugs is replacing in many cases, the use of hard narcotics such as opium, heroin, and cocaine.

The use of these drugs is more and more prevalent among the so-called white collar youth who have never had prior delinquency or criminal records.

The use of these drugs is increasingly identified as a cause of sexual crime.

The ease with which both barbiturates and amphetamines could formerly be obtained legally in the United States was recently dramatized by a television producer. According to Walsh (187) a Columbia Broadcasting System producer set up a fictitious company in Manhattan and through an investment of about $600 was able to obtain from the manufacturers the equivalent of more than 1 million standard tablets, worth between $250,000 and $500,000 in the black market. Nine of the 19 companies from which the drugs were ordered delivered them without asking for proof of licence or Food and Drug Act registration.

Despite opposition from the American Medical Association, the American Pharmaceutical Association, the Pharmaceutical Manufacturers Association, and the National Association of Retail Druggists, the Dodd bill was eventually passed. In the context of this review, the passage of this bill is significant because it indicates the deep concern of the United States government about what it considered to be a serious and widespread problem—amphetamine and barbiturate abuse, a concern scarcely reflected in the pertinent American medical literature.

Medical reports of amphetamine abuse in Canada are practically nil. The only articles found in the Canadian literature were

those of Mitchell and Denton (128) of a fatal case of amphetamine intoxication in a nurse, and of Grantham, *et al.* (76), from
Quebec dealing with psychiatric conditions associated with
amphetamine abuse (*vide supra*, p. 75). In addition Caplan
reported in 1963 (35) a case of severe dependence on various
anorectics in a 27-year-old woman. This included first the use of
phenmetrazine in doses of 75 mg daily for 6 months, of Dexamyl
(*d*-amphetamine 5 mg and amobarbital, 32 mg) in doses of 15
tablets daily for 18 months, and finally diethylpropion in doses of
up to 7500 mg daily! She found the drugs interchangeable and
resorted to one or other depending on their availability.

Despite the scarcity of medical reports the legislators and the
press have periodically emphasized the widespread abuse of
amphetamines and of barbiturates in this country. In September,
1961, the Canadian government enacted Part III of the Food and
Drugs Act and Regulations designed to limit the use of what were
called controlled drugs exclusively to medical purposes. The bill
included provisions for the keeping of records by manufacturers,
distributors, pharmacists, and physicians.

Commenting on the effects of the new regulation, R. C. Hammond of the Narcotic Control Division of the Department of
National Health and Welfare stated in July, 1964 (83), that "The
controls have proved effective in reducing the illicit market
although there still remains more to be accomplished." He emphasized that apart from abuse of the drugs by delinquents and
psychopaths, there is widespread abuse, including addiction and
even fatalities, resulting from excessive medical prescription. He
added: "This situation exists to a much greater extent than many
physicians realize." He also called attention to the extensive prescribing of methamphetamine as an appetite suppressant and
remarked that "there is strong evidence that the addiction poten-
tialities of this drug are not fully realized and appreciated". He
stressed the responsibility of physicians in dealing with these
problems.

According to Hammond (84) amphetamines and barbiturates
are not produced in Canada. The drugs are imported in bulk
either in powder or as finished pharmaceutical products by
licensed dealers. Imports of amphetamines during 1962 amounted

118

to 424 kg, which would be equivalent to 84,800,000 5-mg tablets, or approximately 4.5 tablets per year for every man, woman, and child in the country. This rough estimate would indicate that the consumption of these drugs in Canada is substantially lower than that in the United States, where it was estimated in 1958 to amount to about 20 tablets per capita.

SUMMARY

The terms "addiction" and "habituation," as applied to drugs, have undergone several revisions of definition by the Expert Committee of the World Health Organization. The main point of differentiation between them has been the presence of physical dependence and withdrawal symptoms in true addiction. In practice the terms have proven extremely difficult to apply in relation to amphetamines and certain other drugs. For this and other reasons the Expert Committee has recently recommended the replacement of the two terms by the single term "drug dependence," with the drug type specified.

Review of the literature indicates a sharp difference of opinion with respect to whether or not the amphetamines can produce addiction as originally defined. Those who do not believe in the existence of amphetamine addiction stress: (1) the small number of cases reported; (2) the virtual absence of "pure" amphetamine abuse, most cases also using other drugs to excess; (3) the claimed absence of physical withdrawal symptoms; and (4) the fact that the individuals concerned are usually psychopaths. Those who do believe that amphetamine addiction occurs have emphasized: (1) that the apparent scarcity of cases is due mainly to missed diagnoses, even in extreme cases such as amphetamine psychosis; (2) that physical withdrawal symptoms are demonstrable by the use of modern electrophysiological techniques; (3) that abnormal personality types are common among addicts to all drugs and not only to amphetamines, and in addition some amphetamine addicts had normal pre-addiction personalities; and (4) that the intense craving for amphetamines gives rise to serious damage to both the individual and society at large.

Review of the literature has shown many case reports of chronic amphetamine abuse, that is, an inability to do without the drug for reasons other than legitimate medical indications. These patients, regardless of whether or not they developed a toxic psychosis, had certain features in common, which are illustrated by six typical case histories. All of them suffered periodic or chronic states of intoxication, with the usual signs of central nervous system overstimulation and sometimes sympathetic overactivity. Many had anorexia, insomnia, irritability, and erratic behavior. Abuse of other drugs was common, especially barbiturates which were taken to counteract the insomnia. Development of tolerance was common, and often marked, and the problems of obtaining the large doses required led in many cases to financial hardship, neglect of family, and antisocial behavior such as theft and forgery of prescriptions. In addition, physical dependence has been indicated recently by the discovery of certain abnormal electroencephalographic and electro-oculographic patterns during amphetamine withdrawal, which are abolished immediately by restoring the drug. It is possible that the absence of severe withdrawal symptoms is related to the relatively low rate of elimination of the drug. It is therefore concluded that addiction to amphetamines does occur.

Experience in various countries is reviewed. In the postwar period Japan has had a problem of epidemic proportions. The characteristics of amphetamine abuse in Japan are essentially the same as those already described, and the reasons for the unusually large dimensions of the problem appear to be the ready availability of the drugs and the breakdown in social morale following the country's defeat.

In recent years there has been an apparent increase in the frequency of abuse of amphetamines and related substances in the United Kingdom. Most of the earlier reports dealt with men admitted to psychiatric hospitals because of amphetamine psychoses. More recently there has been increasing concern over the number of neurotic and depressed housewives who often begin using the drugs on medical prescription, and of thrill-seeking teenagers who obtain the drugs illegally. The characteristics of the female addicts were essentially the same as those already described. In contrast, most of the teenage users did not appear to be dependent upon the drugs, using them only on weekends and in a specific social setting.

Except for a few recent reports of sizable series of amphetamine psychoses the American medical literature contains very little reference to problems of amphetamine abuse. Despite this, federal government agencies uncovered sufficient evidence of widespread illicit sales and drug abuse to justify the introduction of restrictive legislation within the past year. The situation in Canada appears to be essentially the same, although the total *per capita* use of amphetamines is less than that in the United States.

VI. Abuse of Amphetamine-like Drugs

DURING THE PAST 10 YEARS several new drugs, recommended mainly as appetite suppressants have been introduced. They include phenmetrazine, phendimetrazine, phenyl-*tert*-butylamine resin, benzphetamine, and diethylpropion. These compounds are chemically and pharmacologically closely related to amphetamine.

The mechanism by which these drugs produce their anorexigenic effect is not known with certainty. Modell (129) is of the opinion that it is probably based on their stimulating effect on the central nervous system rather than on any primary effect on appetite, and that their mechanism of action in this respect is the same as that of the amphetamines proper. He considers that none of them is a true central appetite depressant but that they act by distracting the patient's abnormal drive for food through the sense of well-being that they produce. For these reasons, he refers to the whole group as "central-stimulating appetite distractors" and considers that the risk of unpleasant central and peripheral effects, serious poisoning, tolerance, and habituation cannot be ruled out with these newer drugs without extensive clinical experience.

Two other drugs related to the amphetamines—pipradrol and methylphenidate—have been introduced primarily for use as anti-depressants. Their anorexigenic and peripheral sympathomimetic effects are minimal, relative to their central stimulatory action, but do occur occasionally in susceptible individuals. Although an extensive review of the literature of these newer drugs was not carried out, several references were found in the course of this work that amply substantiate Modell's contentions concerning their risks. This is particularly true with respect to the development of addiction to phenmetrazine with resulting psychotic reactions in many instances. This is not surprising since phenmetrazine is the oldest of these drugs, having been introduced in 1954. Cases of abuse of methylphenidate and of diethyl-propion, introduced more recently, have also been reported.

PHENMETRAZINE ABUSE

General information concerning cases of phenmetrazine abuse, found incidentally during the survey of the amphetamine literature, is summarized in Table XIII. It is interesting to note that 43 of the 45 patients were women and that with two exceptions they were all young, their ages ranging from 14 to 39 years. The reason for this is not clear. Abely, *et al.* (2), who reported having seen 15 cases in a period of three years, referred to all of them as instances of hyperorexia in single young women more or less sexually frustrated and concerned with their appearance. Excessive appetite would lead to obesity and this in turn to the use of anorectics. On the other hand, in the 12 cases reported by Evans obesity was the original reason for taking phenmetrazine in only 2, the remainder having resorted to it for its stimulant properties.

The data presented in Table XIII, and especially the examination of the following individual case histories, clearly show that the central stimulating effects of phenmetrazine in appropriate doses are indistinguishable from those of the classic amphetamines. Twelve of the 28 cases for which individual information was available had abused amphetamines in the past. They then resorted to phenmetrazine either because it was prescribed to them as an alternative to amphetamines, or because phenmetrazine could be obtained without prescription while amphetamines could not. The general features of the development of dependence to phenmetrazine, including the production of psychotic reactions, are so strikingly similar to those of the amphetamines that they require no special discussion. A few case histories will illustrate the point.

Case Histories

CASE 1. Bethell (25) described the case of a 29-year-old woman of psychopathic personality who suddenly began to complain that the floor was magnetized and her jewellery electrified. When she was admitted to hospital three days later she was "dishevelled, tense,

TABLE XIII

REPORTED CASES OF PHENMETRAZINE ABUSE

Author	Reference	Sex	Age	Maximum daily dose	Duration of use	Psychotic reactions	Previous abuse of amphetamine	Other drugs taken to excess
Bethell (1957) U.K.	25	F	29	400 mg	3 mo.	x	x	
Clein (1957) U.K.	40	F	31	1500 mg	10 mo.			alcohol
Glatt (1957) U.K.	73	M	35	1750 mg	4 mo.	x	x	alcohol; barbiturates
Seager & Foster (1958) U.K.	163	F	23	1500 mg	?			
		F	27	250 mg	18 mo.		x	
Dewar & MacCammond (1959) U.K.	55	F	?	750 mg	1 wk.	x		
Silverman (1959) U.K.	167	F	23	500 mg	18 mo.	x		
Evans (1959) U.K.	59	F	33	1500 mg	3 yr.	x	x	alcohol
		F	26	500 mg	3 yr.	x	x	alcohol; barbiturates; Persomnia
		F	31	500 mg	4 mo.	x	x	
		F	33	1500 mg	1 yr.	x		
		F	33	400 mg	4 wk.	x	x	
		M	19	125 mg	6 days	x		alcohol
		F	51	1000 mg	2 yr.	x		
		F	24	500 mg	18 mo.	x	x	alcohol
		F	24	1000 mg	18 mo.	x		
		F	28	100 mg	2 yr.	x		
		F	26	1000 mg	18 mo.	x	x	aspirin; marihuana
		M	26	1000 mg	4 mo.	x		
Rosen & Oberman (1960) U.S.A.	154	F	23	750 mg	1 yr.		x	
Abely, et al. (1960) France	1	F	23	250 mg	4 yr.	x		alcohol
		F	28	1000 mg	2 yr.	x		
Darling (1961) U.S.A.	51	F	?	500 mg	9 mo.		x	alcohol
Schulz (1961) Germany	161	F	42	100 mg	years	x		sedatives
		F	39	250 mg	2 yr.	x		
		F	24	?	?	x		alcohol
		F	29	1 "package"	6 yr.	x		alcohol; Tradon
Welsh (1962) U.S.A.	191	F	14	?	2 yr.			
Oswald & Thacore (1963) U.K.	137	2 cases (females) No individual data given						
Abely, et al. (1963) France	2	15 cases (females) No individual data given						

depressed and emotional, but otherwise there were no abnormal findings." She was given chlorpromazine and calmed down in a few days. For 3 months prior to admission she had become increasingly irritable, suspicious, restless at night, and unduly fearful of burglars. She had taken at least 1400 tablets of phenmetrazine during the 12 weeks prior to admission, and noted that 12 phenmetrazine tablets gave the same effect as that of "a few" *d*-amphetamine tablets. She had switched to phenmetrazine when her father asked the nearby druggist to stop supplying her with *d*-amphetamine. Her reason for taking the drug was "to forget everything and to be able to go off and enjoy herself with her friends."

CASE 2. Evans (59) reported the case of a 26-year-old single woman journalist who, after 6 years of taking 6 tablets of amphetamine sulfate per day, resorted to phenmetrazine which she took for 3 years. She generally consumed 10 to 15 tablets daily, but after a love affair was broken off 6 months before admission she became seriously depressed and temporarily took up to 20 tablets daily. During this time she developed paranoid delusions and ideas of reference, as well as auditory and visual hallucinations. On admission she was fully cooperative and cheerful, her speech was normal, and she claimed insight into her delusions, attributing them to her abuse of phenmetrazine. Later she became impulsive and overactive, attacking a member of the staff. Her hallucinations and delusions re-appeared; she felt that she was going to be brainwashed and converted to communism, that her doctor was hypnotizing her, and so forth. There was slight pressure of talk, emotional lability and elation, but no disorientation. After 3 months she appeared free of psychotic symptoms.

CASE 3. Abely, *et al.* (1), described a case of phenmetrazine abuse in a 23-year-old woman who had been consuming 125 to 250 mg daily for 4 years because of a strong fear of putting on weight. She gradually became nervous, impatient, sometimes aggressive, and suffered from insomnia. She had had 2 psychotic episodes, and had been hospitalized and given insulin-shock therapy. She recovered temporarily, but went back to the abuse of phenmetrazine and to her bizarre behavior. On admission she showed mental automatism, ideas of influence and of physical danger, grimaces, verbal stereotypy, disorientation, cyanosis of the limbs, absence of abdominal reflexes, and dysmenorrhea. Nevertheless, her affect was normal and communication was reasonably good. The patient recovered almost completely in about 2 months, the treatment consisting of sedatives and vitamins.

The comments of Evans (59) with respect to the characteristics of phenmetrazine abuse are of interest, since his series of 16 patients was the largest, and included 12 who suffered psychotic disturbances. He considered that the 12 patients who developed psychosis could be divided into two groups. The first included 7 patients whose symptoms were indistinguishable from those of an amphetamine psychosis and who recovered within a week of stopping the drug. Four of them had relapses when they resorted to phenmetrazine again. He concluded that: "The history of excessive intake of preludin, a frank psychosis and its rapid resolution on stopping the drug, justifies the term psychosis due to preludin." The second group of 5 patients required 5 to 12 weeks to recover. Their symptoms differed slightly from those of the first group. Two patients were elated and more active, and another 2 had definite schizophrenic thought disorder, with vagueness, overinclusiveness, and bizarre associations. Evans considered it possible that in these patients a psychosis coincided by chance with the taking of phenmetrazine, that the patients took the drug to alleviate early symptoms of psychosis, that they continued taking phenmetrazine while under observation, or that large doses of phenmetrazine can cause a schizophrenic type of illness lasting weeks or months.

The group as a whole resembled other drug addicts in several respects. All but one were single or divorced; 13 had an unstable work record; 13 had previously taken alcohol, other drugs, or amphetamines; 5 had a severely disturbed upbringing; none had paranoid traits when well; and 4 were extroverts. Characteristically, some of the patients first denied taking the drug, or minimized the doses. Some had originally taken the drug to reduce, subsequently noticing the stimulant effect. In Evans's words: "This may account for the preponderance of females." Others had taken it primarily as a stimulant. Tolerance developed in all the patients and with 2 exceptions, they all took more than 10 tablets a day for many weeks. Withdrawal symptoms were not common, but 4 patients showed depression and marked lethargy for several days, and one patient had lability of mood. Although only 2 patients demanded the drug while in hospital, they found it difficult to abstain after discharge.

The differential diagnosis presents the same problems as that of amphetamine psychosis since the clinical condition resembles paranoid schizophrenia and cannot be distinguished from amphetamine or bromide psychosis, or from alcoholic hallucinosis. In addition, no tests for phenmetrazine in the urine are at present available, so that the diagnosis depends primarily on the history of phenmetrazine abuse and on rapid recovery after withdrawal.

The similarities between the characteristics and consequences of amphetamine and phenmetrazine abuse should be obvious from this review. From the point of view of the properties of phenmetrazine that make it susceptible of chronic abuse—mainly its central stimulating effect—there is little to distinguish it from the amphetamines proper. Chronic abusers of phenmetrazine generally reach higher doses (Table XIII) than abusers of amphetamine do, probably because phenmetrazine is a less potent stimulating agent. This difference is also true of the recommended therapeutic doses: d-amphetamine sulphate, 5 to 15 mg; amphetamine sulphate, 10 to 30 mg; and phenmetrazine, 25 to 75 mg. The statements of the manufacturers (180) that "Preludin is a safe anorexigenic agent. . . ," that "Preludin produces virtually no mental stimulation yet sufficient mild elevation of mood to pleasantly counteract the depression and lassitude often caused by a low caloric intake," that it has "exceptional safety and strikingly low incidence of side effects. . . ," and that ". . . there have been no reports of significant toxic reactions to Preludin. . . ." seem at best misleading.

Since this review is not complete, definite conclusions with respect to the incidence of phenmetrazine abuse are not possible. However, two observations seem permissible. Firstly, 21 of the 45 cases listed in Table XIII were reported from Great Britain. This is in keeping with the high incidence of amphetamine abuse reported in that country in recent years. Secondly, 12 of those cases, in addition to another 4 not listed in Table XIII, were seen by one author in a period of six months. In Evans's own words: "I supposed the condition to be rare, but within six months I saw no fewer than sixteen patients who had taken preludin and had become ill." It is interesting to note that Evans, like Connell, carried on this work at the Maudsley Hospital in London and his paper appeared a year after the publication of Connell's *Amphetamine Psychosis*. This suggests, once more, that a realistic estimate of the incidence of this type of drug abuse depends on the

127

full awareness of its existence and characteristics, leading to a correct diagnosis. This does not appear to have been widely enough recognized.

METHYLPHENIDATE ABUSE

In 1963 McCormick and McNeel (127a) reviewed the literature on abuse of methylphenidate and reported an original case. This was a 41-year-old divorced man who had been an alcoholic for 20 years. Six months prior to his admission to hospital he had had methylphenidate prescribed, in a dosage of 40 to 60 mg per day, for the treatment of his alcoholism. He took the drug parenterally and soon increased the dose to 100 to 200 mg per day. A few weeks later he developed paranoid delusions, involving fears of spies and of being killed, which became so severe that he was unable to leave his home and had to be hospitalized. On admission he was hyperactive, confused, fearful, and delusional, and had visual hallucinations involving "evil signs" on walls, and objects floating in the air. The physical examination was negative. Withdrawal of methylphenidate and administration of anticonvulsants, sedatives, chlorpromazine, and fluid and nutritional supplements led to a gradual clearing of confusion and to a diminution of the fears and agitation. The patient continued to show some ideas of reference and disorganized thinking during his 24-day period of hospitalization. During this time he was known to have obtained the drug surreptitiously at least once. He left the hospital against medical advice.

McCormick and McNeel felt that although this psychotic reaction might have been "purely incidental" to the abuse of methylphenidate it was "so similar to the toxicomania seen with amphetamine abuse that the relationship to the drug is most suggestive." They also stressed that the type of reaction "is probably determined by the premorbid personality rather than by the pharmacologic action of the drug."

Their review of the pertinent literature indicates that at least 12 other cases of methylphenidate abuse have been reported and variously labelled as "addiction," "borderline" addiction, or

128

"questionable" addiction, suggesting again a similarity with the questions posed by the abuse of amphetamines.

DIETHYLPROPION ABUSE

Although only 4 cases of abuse of diethylpropion were found in the literature, the story is much the same as with the other stimulants, including the fact that all cases had previously abused amphetamines, phenmetrazine, or both.

Clein and Benady (41) reported in 1962 on a 26-year-old single woman who was admitted to hospital on 4 occasions during a 16-month period with paranoid delusions and auditory hallucinations. On the first admission she was diagnosed as schizophrenic. On all occasions she improved in a matter of weeks. During the fourth stay in hospital it was established that she had been taking 9 to 90 tablets (225 to 2250 mg) daily of diethylpropion, and this was confirmed by her father. She had been taking first *d*-amphetamine and then phenmetrazine from age 15, and at age 24 had switched to diethylpropion because it was more easily obtainable. She was a woman of inadequate personality with marked inferiority feelings who stated that diethylpropion gave her courage and made her feel more lively. In the authors' opinion the patient's psychotic symptoms were similar in every respect to those seen in amphetamine psychosis. They further stated: "It seems that certain vulnerable people with inadequate and psychopathic personalities may become habituated and addicted to almost any drug which has a euphoriant action, no matter how slight that action is, and will go out of their way to obtain such drugs in large quantities to get the stimulation they crave."

In 1962 Kuenssberg (111) reported two cases seen over a 3-week period. A 32-year-old married woman had been taking 75 to 150 mg of diethylpropion daily for 3 months to lose weight. She lost 18 pounds but was still overweight. She developed "a most remarkable change in personality," with inability to concentrate, suspiciousness, hyperexcitability, and emotionality. "These psychotic symptoms were undoubtedly caused by diethylpropion, as its withdrawal reestablished her previous competent, generous personality." Her health had been excellent for the past 20 years, except for early psychotic symptoms 5 years previously caused by d-amphetamine. The second case was that of a 38-year-old married woman who took undetermined amounts of diethylpropion (probably 4 times the normal dose) on her own and developed a severe psychotic state requiring hospitalization. She was supposed to have been successfully cured of her previous addiction to d-amphetamine.

Kuenssberg (112) further reported that in the British black market a single tablet of diethylpropion sells for 1 shilling, yet a whole month's supply for legitimate medical reasons costs 2 shillings. In other instances patients have had the drug sent to them directly from the United States because their doctors were reluctant to continue prescribing it. He concluded: "When a drug becomes an item of self-medication to such an extent, surely the slippery pathway past habituation to addiction has been started."

In 1963 Caplan (35) reported in Canada the case of a 27-year-old married woman who sought psychiatric help because of a state of depression provoked by her inability to meet the cost of her habituation to various central nervous system stimulants. When seen she was tense, agitated, and rather suspicious. She talked rapidly, her mood was labile, she smoked heavily, and her appearance was rather unkempt. Her economic, social, and marital problems were considerable. About 3 years earlier she had become increasingly depressed and begun to overeat, her weight rising from 128 to 152 pounds. A friend gave her phenmetrazine and she was delighted to discover that it gave her a "lift." She took 75 mg daily for 6 months until her doctor refused further prescriptions. She then switched to Dexamyl (a mixture of d-amphetamine 5 mg and amobarbital 32 mg per tablet) which she obtained without prescription. She took 15 tablets daily for 18 months. When unable to obtain the drugs she had periods of deep depression and was hospitalized twice within one year when she threatened to commit suicide. She then discovered that diethylpropion could be obtained without prescription and began taking 1125 mg daily, gradually increasing the dose to a maximum of 7500 mg daily. On this dosage she had insomnia and anorexia —she lost 24 pounds—but felt sure she could cope with anything.

Without the drug she was jumpy, nervous, depressed, weeping, seclusive, had ideas of reference, and feared open spaces. The cost of the drug, amounting to about $7.25 per 100 tablets (or about $21 per day) led to financial and social distress. After one month of supportive treatment with non-barbiturate nocturnal sedation she felt considerably better, but the urge for the drug remained.

The manufacturers of diethylpropion state (181) that "Tenuate is a totally different anorexic agent, virtually free of central nervous system stimulation, for any patient whose weight must come down." In addition, one of their representatives, in a letter to the *British Medical Journal* (151), took exception to the statement by Oswald and Thacore (137) that amphetamines, phenmetrazine, "and drugs with comparable actions, such as diethylpropion, are dangerous drugs in fact, if not yet in law." He considered this a "sweeping generalization" since it was based on one reported case of abuse of diethylpropion in an emotionally disturbed individual while hundreds of millions of tablets of the drug had been prescribed. In his opinion: "The weight of presently available evidence indicates that the amphetamines, phenmetrazine, and diethylpropion hydrochloride are safe, effective, and useful when given under proper medical supervision according to the manufacturers' directions. The occasional report of addiction for these, or indeed for any compound, has much wider implications than merely the nature of the chemical substance involved. Certainly the sociological and psychological considerations should not be neglected." He further considered that "If the compound were indeed addictive and dangerous, reports of this kind would occur with much greater frequency than this."

Despite these claims it appears obvious from the evidence here reviewed that diethylpropion, or any drug with central stimulating properties, has the same potential for abuse as the amphetamines. That the individuals who do abuse these drugs are emotionally disturbed or addiction prone, or possess psychopathic or inadequate personalities, cannot be used as an argument to exonerate the drugs, since it takes both a drug and a susceptible subject to produce addiction or milder degrees of dependency. Besides, these same individuals do not abuse a large number of other drugs that are equally available to them but lack the effects which they seek. Finally, the argument so frequently used, that scarcity of reports indicates absence of abuse has been amply demonstrated throughout this review to be unfounded.

SUMMARY

A number of newer drugs, including phenmetrazine and diethylpropion, are widely used (often without medical prescription) for the treatment of obesity. These drugs are closely related, both chemically and pharmacologically, to the amphetamines. Numerous cases of drug abuse, including many which have resulted in toxic psychoses, show clinical characteristics which are indistinguishable from those of amphetamine abuse. In fact, many of the patients had previously abused amphetamines. As with amphetamine addiction and psychosis, awareness of the problem in relation to these drugs appears to result in much greater frequency of diagnosis than is otherwise the case. Similar pictures have resulted from the abuse of methylphenidate, an amphetamine-like drug with minimal peripheral sympathomimetic effect, which is used principally as a stimulant and antidepressant agent. It is evident that a variety of stimulant and mood elevating drugs may be abused and may give rise in extreme cases to similar psychotic reactions.

VII. Social Significance of
Amphetamine Abuse

THIS SURVEY OF THE LITERATURE on the toxic and other undesirable effects of the amphetamines has shown that these drugs can produce:

1. Acute toxic states characterized by symptoms of overstimulation of the sympathetic and central nervous systems. The severity of the symptoms depends on the dose and on the susceptibility of the individual and can range from mild states of excitation through acute psychotic reactions of a paranoid type to death. These toxic reactions are not infrequent in young children having access to the drugs in their homes.

2. Various degrees of dependence ranging from mild habituation to strong compulsion to using the drugs chronically. The more severe cases of dependence show all the characteristics of true addiction.

3. The development of marked tolerance leading to the need for increasing doses, with marked chronic undesirable effects such as insomnia, anorexia, and abnormal behavior.

4. The development of transitory psychotic reactions clinically indistinguishable from paranoid schizophrenia. These toxic psychoses can occur both as a result of a single dose of amphetamines and in chronic users of the drugs. In the latter the prognosis is bad in the sense that the risk of recurrence is directly related to the continued consumption of amphetamines.

5. Damage to society in the form of neglect of family and work, financial irresponsibility, crime, and other antisocial behavior.

Many of the problems posed by the use and abuse of the amphetamines and similar drugs are particular instances of larger problems in relation to the use of any drug capable of altering man's mood. Indeed these problems are much broader in that they include, as well, the use and abuse of alcohol and various naturally occurring psychotropic agents. The latter substances (alcoholic beverages, tea, coffee, marihuana, coca, and khat, for example) cannot be considered drugs in the strict sense of the term, since they are not usually consumed for medicinal purposes, but as integral parts of various cultures. This distinction is of importance in the sense that it influences to a very large extent the manner in which society judges the relative merits and liabilities of the psychotropic drugs on the one hand and the natural substances on the other, and the restrictions that it imposes upon their respective uses.

There are many parallels between the use of alcohol and the non-medical use of amphetamines, including the fact that although large numbers of individuals resort to these agents to feel better, or at least different, only a small proportion become dependent to the extent that harmful effects result. But, from the point of view of society, there is a major difference: generally speaking, the use of amphetamines for non-medical purposes is not an accepted form of social behavior. Therefore, the evaluation of the untoward effects of the amphetamines, including their indiscriminate use by the lay public, has been based throughout this review on the fact that these substances are drugs rather than part of the common fare of human beings, and on the related assumption that their use should be limited to medical purposes exclusively. A discussion of the merits or otherwise of the use of the drugs by society at large for other purposes, such as the production of an increased feeling of well-being or for the enhancement of performance, is beyond the scope of this work.

The distinction, however, between drugs and naturally occurring chemical agents with similar properties is not always easy to make. The use of amphetamines for non-medical purposes, and the habit of chewing khat leaves prevalent in certain countries of the Middle East and eastern Africa, offer an interesting example in this respect.

Khat (*Catha edulis*) is a bush which originated in Arabia but which also grows spontaneously in eastern Africa (115). The inhabitants of these regions, including Saudi Arabia, Yemen, Aden, Somalia, Ethiopia, Eritrea, and Kenya, as well as Afghanistan, have

134

long been in the habit of chewing the fresh leaves of the bush. The habit is social rather than solitary, and is usually indulged in by the men after work hours. They sit about in groups chewing khat, smoking, and drinking tea, soft drinks, and even alcohol. At first, the khat-chewer experiences a feeling of well-being with diminution of fatigue, hunger, and worries. As the euphoria changes into hypomania, thought processes are speeded up, talkativeness and aggressiveness appear, and later there is inability to concentrate. There is also sexual excitation ending in spontaneous ejaculation without orgasm. Physically there is mydriasis, tachycardia, and hypertension. As the stimulating effects of khat wane, they are followed by depression with general fatigue, intense thirst, anorexia, and insomnia. The active principle presumably responsible for these effects is the alkaloid cathine or d-nor-isoephedrine. In addition to cathine, two amorphous alkaloids, cathinine and cathidine, as well as substantial amounts of tannins, have also been extracted from the plant. The chemical and pharmacological similarities between cathine and the amphetamines are striking, although cathine appears to be less potent (196).

According to Laurent (115) the need for khat is not insurmountable, but its habitual use can lead to the following medical and social consequences: (1) disturbances of the gastro-intestinal tract such as paralytic ileus, constipation, stomatitis, gastritis, and anorexia leading to multiple nutritional deficiencies; (2) disturbances of the cardiovascular system including meningeal hemorrhages, hemiplegias, cardiac infarction, pulmonary edema, and perhaps some cases of hypertension which is common in these areas; (3) psychiatric disturbances such as intractable insomnia leading to anxiety and irritability; impotence; states of excitation ranging from motor hyperexcitability to manic crises commonly seen in these regions, and confused delusional states, which seem to be the most obvious complication and always occur in highly intoxicated individuals.

In Laurent's opinion the social consequences are even more serious than the untoward effects on the individual. Since 60 to 70 per cent of all adults indulge in the habit, and since its cost amounts to about half of a laborer's wages, there is an important diversion of income to this end. This aggravates still further the nutritional deficiencies which are common in these under-developed countries and leads to an increase in morbidity, infant mortality, and tuberculosis. Although the problem is still local, faster and better means of communication are responsible for a rapid spread of the use of khat. This was not hitherto possible because the fresh leaves lose their potency within 3 or 4 days. The habit is seen mainly among Moslems and only rarely among Christians, indicating that the choice of drug and extent of its use are functions of social and cultural factors rather than of psychological vulnerability. According to Laurent several measures taken in these areas to curtail the habit, such as partial or total prohibition and high taxes, have failed.

The Expert Committee on Addiction-producing Drugs of the World Health Organization has recently called attention to the problem of khat-chewing in the regions involved and to its similarities to the non-medical uses of amphetamines (196). Indeed, the main difference would appear to be that amphetamines are not an accepted part of our general culture, and their misuse is detrimental mainly to the user and his immediate associates, while khat is a normal ingredient of Middle Eastern culture and causes widespread harm to the whole society.

The khat problem makes clear therefore that, while a society may incorporate the widespread use of naturally occurring stimulants into its culture, it may none the less suffer serious consequences. If the non-medical use of amphetamines were to become a generally accepted form of behavior in our society the results might well be the same. By and large, the cases of amphetamine dependence discussed in this review are instances of individual and socially concealed abuse of the drugs. These cases are significant mainly with respect to the consequences to the individual. On the other hand, the epidemic proportions of amphetamine abuse in Japan and the current abuse of amphetamines and other drugs among teenagers in Britain show that when the use of these stimulants becomes established as part of a subculture it gives rise to broad and possibly intractable problems. Once such a pattern becomes established, measures to curtail it may well be ineffectual, as evidenced by the history of Prohibition on this continent. It is therefore of great importance to know how widespread the abuse of amphetamines is in our society, and whether or not it is becoming a behavioral norm among certain sub-cultures.

This question cannot be adequately answered from the data available. But, since there are strong suggestions that amphetamines and amphetamine-like substances are abused by various sectors of society, research specifically designed to establish the true extent of this type of drug abuse is most desirable.

The following research projects would contribute substantially to the clarification of this question:

1. A survey designed to find out the actual amounts of amphetamines and amphetamine-like substances prescribed in a large urban center and the purposes for which they are prescribed.

2. A follow-up study, with the collaboration of general practitioners and pharmacists, of obese patients who have been treated with the drugs, in order to find out how many, if any, become dependent and continue to take them on their own initiative.

3. A study of the incidence of amphetamine psychosis. This could be done in collaboration with psychiatric hospitals by performing tests for amphetamine-like substances in the urines of all patients admitted with a picture of paranoid schizophrenia, and by correlating the results of such tests with the histories of the patients and with the course of the illness.

4. A study of the incidence of amphetamine abuse in all patients admitted to the clinics of a large alcoholism treatment center such as the Alcoholism and Drug Addiction Research Foundation of Ontario. This would also involve urine tests for amphetamines on all admissions.

5. A study of the use of amphetamines at examination time in a group of university students.

6. A study of the incidence of amphetamine consumption by delinquent juveniles. This could be done by performing urine tests for amphetamines immediately upon arrest, perhaps with the collaboration of a government crime detection laboratory.

From projects such as these it should be possible to derive the information which would remove the question of amphetamine abuse from the realm of conjecture and permit a sound appraisal of its present and potential significance in our society.

APPENDICES

A. An Overview of Recent Developments

DURING THE 1960s there occurred an explosive increase in the non-medical use of amphetamines, especially in North America (1, 11, 18, 30, 33, 38) and in some parts of Europe (4, 35). This was part of the more general increase in the consumption of a variety of psychoactive drugs. Most North American surveys during this period showed that the extent of use of amphetamines, particularly by late teenagers and young adults, was exceeded only by that of alcohol, tobacco, and marihuana (5, 36). In other countries, such as Sweden (4, 17, 35) and Czechoslovakia (42), phenmetrazine is claimed to be the major drug used for non-medical purposes. A short-lived epidemic of intravenous use of methamphetamine also took place in England in 1968 (19, 21).

The problems arising from the non-medical use of amphetamines and related drugs by adults in the general population, of the type described in the body of this monograph, have continued. Indeed during the last few years there have been reports of such cases from countries where the problem had not previously been noted (3, 22, 25, 26, 42). However, the newer pattern of amphetamine use differs from that described in the text in at least three important respects: a preference for the intravenous route of administration, a tendency for young users to share their drug experiences in "speed" pads or communities, and the epidemic nature of the phenomenon. The specific implications of some of these features are discussed in Appendices B and C.

The difference in pattern has led many observers to consider the problem as quite different from that outlined in the body of this monograph. Frequent reference is made to the picture of high-dose intravenous use *as opposed to* low-dose oral use. Indeed one recent report stated that the earlier literature was "of little value [to physicians treating "speed" users] in that it dealt primarily with low-dose oral patterns" (40). This misconception is dealt

141

with in Appendix B. Undoubtedly the use of the intravenous route of administration introduces specific additional complications. As discussed in the next two appendices, these include the rapidity and intensity of the onset of drug effect, and hence the rate and strength of development of psychological dependence, and also the occurrence of physical complications related to the practice of injection. However, the basic problems are common to both methods of intake and the same individual may use both (34). Fundamentally, amphetamine dependence and its concomitant behavioral and psychiatric complications can develop in comparable manner, regardless of the mode of intake and of the age, social status, and life style of the user. The situation is quite comparable to that found in alcoholism: the drinking patterns may vary widely from periodic binges to the less conspicuous form of steady daily intake of large amounts, yet the basic problems are essentially the same.

North American "speed" users, as described in Appendix C, are generally associated with a recognizable deviant subculture. Although there were earlier indications of this pattern of use in the United States, the phenomenon did not become widespread and highly visible until the late 1960s (18, 24, 30). This occurred in many large urban centers but was particularly evident on the west coast of the United States (9, 12), including the Haight-Ashbury area of San Francisco (33, 34, 37, 38, 40). Here to some extent amphetamine displaced hallucinogens, which had generally been favored by the earlier hippies. "Speed" users share with their Japanese predecessors of nearly two decades earlier, their English counterparts of the early 1960s, and their Swedish contemporaries, their youth, their alienation from society, their clannish behavior, and, of course, many of the complications attendant upon amphetamine use. The absolute numbers of people involved in these outbreaks of amphetamine use cannot be documented accurately. However, the general impression gained from published estimates is that the Japanese epidemic was by far the largest.

Of the three distinguishing features cited above, the least explored and yet the most important from the public health point of view is the epidemic nature of recent patterns of amphetamine use. This is neither new, nor peculiar to the use of stimulants. Drug epidemics of various types have come and gone in the past (6) and, at present, involve other drugs as well. However, there is a clear need for information to explain changes in the social pattern of use of specific drugs. Why was there an amphetamine epidemic in Japan between 1945 and 1955 and not elsewhere? Why, after nearly 40 years of relatively stable levels of use among the general population in North America, did a specific pattern attached to an identifiable subculture become an epidemic problem? Why has phenmetrazine been the equivalent drug of choice in Sweden, and why did this not occur on a comparable scale in other Scandinavian countries? Why is most of the amphetamine used intravenously in North America obtained from illicit manufacturers whereas in other parts of the world it is obtained indirectly from the pharmaceutical industry?

The answers to these and other questions are essential for an understanding of the dynamics of drug epidemics. Brill (6) and Bejerot (4), among others, have dealt with this important question. In general, however, there is a regrettable lack of systematic research on this extremely important topic. Without it, attempts at controlling and preventing future epidemics will inevitably be limited to hit-and-miss measures taken in response to local problems.

During this period there has been constant reassessment of the therapeutic value of the amphetamines and related substances in clinical medicine, particularly their wide use as anorexiants in the control of obesity. A growing consensus that they are of little value, except in narcolepsy and juvenile hyperkinesia, has led to a sharp decrease in the extent of their use (2, 8) and to their prohibition in some parts of the world. The continuing importance of problems of non-medical use of these drugs, despite the change in medical and legal practices, emphasizes the value of understanding the underlying epidemiological process.

A review of the literature published to the end of 1971 on the topics discussed in this monograph reveals that about 400 additional titles have appeared since the publication of the first edition. A sharp rise in the number of publications per year occurred in 1968 and has been maintained since. The main areas researched are sociological problems related to amphetamine and other drug use, medical and psychiatric complications, and the question of amphetamine dependence, including experimental work on self-administration of stimulants by animals. The handful of reports on fatalities associated with amphetamine use (10, 14, 15, 27, 39, 44) reflects the relatively unfounded near-panic that led the communications media, and even some experts in the drug field, to take literally the slogan "speed kills." Though there is some evidence that the mortality rates among those using stimulants intravenously may be higher than in an age-matched population, the difference is not spectacular (20).

There has been very little research on methods of treatment of amphetamine dependence. In view of the apparently intractable nature of this type of drug dependence and of the seriousness of the behavioral and medical complications, research on prevention and treatment are urgently needed, as well as longitudinal studies on the life course of amphetamine addicts.

In the circumstances it would appear profitable and reasonable that workers in this field should be interested in the knowledge and experience of others facing the same problems, regardless of country, culture, or era. An examination of the literature reveals, however, a high degree of parochialism. This applies not only to experience in different countries, but also to the particular drug involved, to patterns of use, and even to scientific and medical disciplines. Despite the similarities between the various national epidemics, each country in turn waited until a local crisis developed before taking the experience of the others seriously. With a few notable exceptions (7, 28) the events in Japan and Sweden were largely ignored until very recently in the English-language literature. Comparable attitudes are reflected in most of the European literature on this subject. Publications dealing with the "speed" question in North America would leave the inexperienced reader with the impression that methamphetamine has clearly distinguishable effects from those of other drugs of the same group. This contention is not supported by observations either in experimental animals (16, 41, 43) or in man (29). Virtually identical descriptions have been given of subjective effects of phenmetrazine by Swedish users (32) and of "speed" by North American

144

users (12). As noted above, the sharp contrast drawn between "low-dose oral" and "high-dose intravenous" use is also unwarranted and misleading.

Regrettably this type of narrow and parochial approach applies even among disciplines. The numerous recent national and international cross-disciplinary symposia on drug use in general and on amphetamine use in particular (13, 31, 35) have to some extent eased these problems. However, if enough physicians and other experts are to achieve sufficient understanding of the various aspects of drug use to lead to the adoption of thoughtful and effective social policies, the large body of knowledge already available must be more widely read and assimilated.

By putting the problems of non-medical use of amphetamines and related drugs in historical and international perspective it is hoped that this monograph will contribute to a better understanding of the field. A comprehensive bibliography dealing with the topics discussed in this volume has also been prepared and is available from the Addiction Research Foundation of Ontario (23).

References

1. ANGRIST, B. M., & GERSHON, S.: Amphetamine abuse in New York City—1966 to 1968, Seminars Psychiat., 1: 195–207, 1969.
2. ANONYMOUS: Freedom from amphetamines, Brit. M. J., iii: 133–4, 1971.
3. ARNOLD, O. H., & HOFMANN, G.: Klinische, psychopathologische und biochemische Untersuchungen an Phenmetrazin-Psychosen, Wien. Ztschr. Nervenh., 27: 294–305, 1969.
4. BEJEROT, N.: Addiction and Society. Springfield, Charles C Thomas, 1970.
5. BERG, D. F.: Illicit Use of Dangerous Drugs in the United States. A Compilation of Studies, Surveys and Polls. U.S. Government Printing Office, Washington, D.C., 1970.
6. BRILL, H.: Recurrent patterns in the history of drugs of dependence and some interpretations. In: Drugs and Youth, ed. by J. R. Wittenborn et al., pp. 8–25. Springfield, Charles C Thomas, 1969.
7. BRILL, H., & HIROSE, T.: The rise and fall of a methamphetamine epidemic: Japan 1945–1955, Seminars Psychiat., 1: 179–92, 1969.
8. CANADIAN MEDICAL ASSOCIATION: Association submits second brief on non-medical use of drugs to LeDain commission, Canad. M.A.J., 104: 738–41, 1971.
9. CAREY, J. T., & MANDEL, J.: A San Francisco Bay Area "speed" scene, J. Health Soc. Behav., 9: 164–74, 1968.
10. CITRON, B. P., HALPERN, M., McCARRON, M., LUNDBERG, G. D., McCORMICK, R., PINCUS, I. J., TATTER, D., & HAVERBACK, B. J.: Necrotizing angiitis associated with drug abuse, New England J. Med., 283: 1003–11, 1970.
11. CLEMENT, W. R., SOLURSH, L. P., & VAN AST, W.: Abuse of amphetamine and amphetamine-like drugs, Psychol. Rep., 26: 343–54, 1970.
12. COHEN, S.: Abuse of centrally stimulating agents among juveniles in California.

In: Abuse of Central Stimulants, ed. by F. Sjoqvist & M. Tottie, pp. 165–85. New York, Raven Press, 1970.

13. COSTA, E., & GARRATINI, S. (eds.): International Symposium on Amphetamines and Related Compounds. New York, Raven Press, 1970.
14. CRAVEY, R. H., & BASELT, R. C.: Methamphetamine poisoning, J. Forensic Sci. Soc., 8: 118–20, 1968.
15. CRAVEY, R. H., & REED, D.: Intravenous amphetamine poisoning—report of three cases, J. Forensic Sci. Soc., 10: 109–12, 1970.
16. DENEAU, G., YANAGITA, R., & SEEVERS, M. H.: Self-administration of psychoactive substances by the monkey. A measure of psychological dependence, Psychopharmacologia, 16: 30–48, 1969.
17. GOLDBERG, L.: Drug abuse in Sweden, Bull. Narcot., 20 (1): 1–31 & (2): 9–36, 1968.
18. GRIFFITH, J.: A study of illicit amphetamine drug traffic in Oklahoma City, Am. J. Psychiat., 123: 560–9, 1966.
19. HAWKS, D., MITCHESON, M., OGBORNE, A., & EDWARDS, G.: Abuse of methylamphetamine, Brit. M.J., ii: 715–21, 1969.
20. INGHE, G.: The present state of abuse and addiction to stimulant drugs in Sweden: In: Abuse of Central Stimulants, ed. by F. Sjoqvist & M. Tottie, pp. 187–214. New York, Raven Press, 1969.
21. JAMES, I. P.: A methamphetamine epidemic? Lancet, i: 916, 1968.
22. JAROSZYNSKI, J., SPASOWICZ, E., & ULASINSKA-RUBACH, D.: Phenetrazine psychoses, Polisk M.J., 10: 253–7, 1971.
23. KALANT, O. J.: Amphetamine Toxicity and Dependence. A Comprehensive Bibliography. Addiction Research Foundation, Toronto, Canada, 1973.
24. KRAMER, J. C., FISCHMAN, V. S., & LITTLEFIELD, D. C.: Amphetamine abuse: pattern and effects of high doses taken intravenously, J.A.M.A., 201: 305–9, 1967.
25. LADEWIG, D., & BATTEGAY, R.: Abuse of anorexics with special reference to newer substances, Int. J. Addict., 6: 167–72, 1971.
26. LADEWIG, D., BATTEGAY, R., & LABHARDT, F.: Stimulantien: Abhängigkeit und Psychosen, Deutsch. Med. Wchnschr., 94: 101–7, 1969.
27. LLOYD, J. T. A., & WALKER, D. R. H.: Death after combined dexamphetamine and phenelzine, Brit. M.J., ii: 168–9, 1965.
28. LOURIA, D. B.: Some aspects of the current drug scene, with emphasis on drugs in use by adolescents, Pediatrics, 42: 904–11, 1968.
29. MARTIN, W. R., SLOAN, J. W., SAPIRA, J. D., & JASINSKI, D. R.: Physiologic, subjective, and behavioral effects of amphetamine, methamphetamine, ephedrine, phenmetrazine, and methylphenidate in man, Clin. Pharmacol. Therap., 12: 245–58, 1971.
30. RAWLIN, J. W.: Street level abusage of amphetamines. In: Amphetamine Abuse, ed. by J. R. Russo. Springfield, Charles C Thomas, 1968.
31. RUSSO, J. R. (ed.): Amphetamine Abuse. Springfield, Charles C Thomas, 1968.
32. RYLANDER, G.: Clinical and medico-criminological aspects of addiction to central stimulating drugs. In Abuse of Central Stimulants, ed. by F. Sjoqvist & M. Tottie, pp. 251–73. New York, Raven Press, 1969.
33. SHICK, J. F. E., SMITH, D. E., & MEYERS, F. H.: Use of amphetamine in the Haight-Ashbury subculture, J. Psychedelic Drugs, 2: 139–71, 1969.
34. SHICK, J. F. E., SMITH, D. E., & MEYERS, F. H.: Patterns of drug use in the Haight-Ashbury neighbourhood, Clin. Toxicol., 3: 19–56, 1970.
35. SJOQVIST, F., & TOTTIE, M. (eds.): Abuse of Central Stimulants. Symposium arranged by the Swedish Committee on International Health Relations, Stockholm, November 25–27, 1968. New York, Raven Press. 1969.
36. SMART, R. G., & FEJER, D.: The extent of illicit drug use in Canada: A review

146

of current epidemiology. In: Critical Issues in Canadian Society, ed. by C. L. Boydell, C. F. Grindstaff, & P. C. Whitehead. Toronto, Holt, Rinehart & Winston, 1971, pp. 508–19.

37. SMITH, D. E.: Speed freaks vs. acid heads—conflict between drug subcultures, Clin. Pediat., 8: 185–8, 1969.
38. SMITH, D. E.: [Medical Staff Conference] Changing drug patterns in the Haight-Ashbury. Calif. Med., 110: 151–7, 1969.
39. SMITH, D. E.: The characteristics of dependence in high-dose methamphetamine abuse, Int. J. Addict., 4: 453–9, 1969.
40. SMITH, D. E., & FISCHER, C. M.: An analysis of 310 cases of acute high-dose methamphetamine toxicity in Haight-Ashbury, Clin. Toxicol., 3: 117–24, 1970.
41. THOMPSON, T., & PICKENS, R.: Stimulant self-administration by animals: some comparisons with opiate self-administration, Fed. Proc., 29: 6–12, 1970.
42. VONDRÁČEK, V., PROKUPEK, J., FISCHER, R., & AHRANBERGOVÁ, M.: Recent patterns of addiction in Czechoslovakia, Brit. J. Psychiat., 114: 285–92, 1968.
43. YANAGITA, T., ANDO, K., & TAKAHASHI, S.: A testing method for psychological dependence liability of drugs in monkeys. In: Committee on Problems of Drug Dependence, Report of the Thirty-Second Meeting, 16–18 Feb. 1970, Washington, D.C., pp. 6583–91.
44. ZALIS, E. G., & PARMLEY, L. F.: Fatal amphetamine poisoning, Arch. Intern. med., 112: 822–6, 1963.

B. The Psychopharmacology of Amphetamine Dependence*

THE STORY of the amphetamines begins in 1887 when Edeleano (13) first synthesized the volatile β-phenylisopropylamine, i.e., amphetamine. These substances are synthetic aromatic amines related both chemically and pharmacologically to a larger group of compounds known as pressor or sympathomimetic amines, such as epinephrine and ephedrine, but having proportionally a greater stimulating effect on the central nervous system. The latter effect, first observed by Alles about 40 years ago (1), is the basis for their therapeutic as well as for their non-medical use. The drugs produce a state of arousal or wakefulness demonstrable both behaviorally (10) and electroencephalographically (7) and accompanied by an increase in psychic and motor activity. This is usually perceived subjectively as a sense of increased energy, mastery, and self-confidence, as faster and more efficient thought and decision-taking, and as a state of well-being or euphoria. Another marked central action of the drugs is appetite inhibition (10). These effects have been the basis for the therapeutic applications (27) of the amphetamines as anti-depressants, in the treatment of narcolepsy, and as anorexiants, as well as for their use during World War II to alleviate fatigue and increase the endurance of the troops. They have also been the basis for the lay, non-medical use of the drugs.

Reports of non-medical use of amphetamines with various medical complications, which appeared in the literature soon after their introduction to clinical medicine, have been extensively assessed in the body of this monograph. They refer for the most

*This appendix is based on the paper by A. E. LeBlanc, O. J. Kalant, and H. Kalant presented on August 18, 1970, at the symposium sponsored by the Council on Drug Abuse in Toronto, Canada.

148

part to isolated instances of chronic oral self-administration of amphetamines. The first reports of non-medical use of amphetamines in epidemic proportions came from Japan in the 1950s (33, 35), but relatively little attention was paid to them in the West until recently (8, 22). However, during the 1960s evidence began to accumulate from Great Britain (6), Sweden (19), and North America (11) which indicated a rapidly increasing spread in the non-medical use of amphetamines and related drugs, particularly among the young. The pattern of use differs significantly from that in earlier reports; there is a preference for the intravenous route of administration (26), and a tendency for users to group themselves into what is referred to as "speed" communities (40).

The question of amphetamine dependence has recently been examined extensively from the sociological (20, 40), psychiatric (14), medical (22), and legal standpoints. However, relatively little attention has been paid to the psychopharmacological features of the drug which are responsible for the development of dependence, and we shall deal primarily with this topic. We believe it to be a very important aspect of the problem, because dependence underlies the heavy regular use of amphetamines, and dependent users are therefore the ones most likely to suffer the most serious effects.

The Expert Committee of the World Health Organization (45) has characterized drug dependence of the amphetamine type in the terms set out on p. 79 of this monograph. Of the features mentioned there, there is no doubt about the existence of tolerance. Leaving aside the question of "speed" there are many well-documented accounts (22) of regular use of doses as high as one gram per day, compared to the normal therapeutic dose of 10 to 30 mg. This cannot be explained in terms of increased metabolism or excretion. Ellison et al. (16) have shown in cats that the tolerance represents a true increase in the ability of the central nervous system to tolerate the effects of the drug, although the mechanism of this adaptation is not clear. On the basis of studies of the distribution of radio-active amphetamine in cats, Siegel et al. (38) contend that tolerance is accompanied by an alteration in the blood-brain barrier, such that the concentration of drug in the brain during the first four hours after administration is less than

149

in non-tolerant animals. However, the difference is small enough that we must still postulate a fundamental increase in tolerance of the brain cells themselves.

It must be noted that the pathways of metabolism of amphetamines are not identical in all species, and the possibility of increased metabolism has not been adequately studied in man (4). An interesting speculation is that the anorexiant effects of amphetamines may affect the drug excretion (26). Renal excretion of amphetamines is markedly influenced by the pH of the urine. Since starvation tends to cause ketosis and a fall in pH of the urine, it would also tend to increase the excretion of amphetamine, and hence the apparent tolerance.

The question of physical dependence is not nearly as well settled. Most writers on this subject agree that there are no serious physical effects of amphetamine withdrawal but emphasize a syndrome of depression, prolonged sleep, and voracious appetite (26, 39). These symptoms have been generally interpreted as the consequence of accumulated fatigue, masked by the drug during the period of its use, and unmasked on withdrawal. It is difficult to explain the increased appetite in these terms since starvation or semi-starvation from other causes is not followed by such abrupt rebound of appetite. The interpretation has probably been clouded by a common tendency to expect all drug withdrawal reactions to resemble those caused by opiates. The report by Smith (39) of "classical withdrawal reactions" implies such a concept. Since many amphetamine users are promiscuous users of other drugs, particularly barbiturates, "classical withdrawal reactions" in a few cases may represent withdrawal from these other drugs. It seems to us more reasonable to consider depression, sleep, and increased appetite as rebound phenomena of physical dependence on stimulant and anorexiant drugs, just as rebound hyperexcitability is an abstinence phenomenon with depressant drugs.

The reports by Oswald and Thacore (34) concerning changes in REM sleep are compatible with this suggestion. Acutely, amphetamine suppresses REM sleep, but with chronic use of the drug this effect is diminished or abolished. On withdrawal of amphetamine there is a marked increase in REM sleep lasting for up to a month, which can be eliminated by renewed administration of the

150

drug. However, it must be noted that the same phenomena have been reported in relation to chronic use of barbiturates and other drugs (24) which produce very different withdrawal pictures from that of amphetamine. Other types of physiological investigation may be more appropriate for demonstrating physical dependence. In our own laboratory we have found that acute administration of amphetamine reduces the startle thresholds in rats (18, 28). On chronic administration the threshold returns to normal, and on withdrawal of amphetamine there is a rebound elevation of threshold. It would be useful to make comparable observations by the method of Bradley and Key (7) of electrical thresholds for electroencephalographic arousal by stimulation of the reticular activating system.

Another factor to be taken into account in considering the relative lack of severity of the amphetamine withdrawal reaction is the quantitative relation between the speed of elimination of the drug and the speed with which the nervous system adapts to this elimination. If the drug is removed slowly, the nervous system is more likely to be able to adapt at a commensurate rate so that little or no withdrawal disturbance is manifest. Abrupt removal of the drug, on the contrary, will reveal physical dependence much more clearly. The ideal example is provided by nalorphine, which displaces morphine from its receptors in the brain and other tissues, producing an almost immediate morphine withdrawal reaction. No analogous compound exists for amphetamines, but rapid elimination by acidification of the urine with ammonium chloride might be a useful way of exaggerating withdrawal effects for experimental study.

Despite the uncertainties concerning physical dependence on amphetamines the essential feature of any drug dependence is psychological dependence, i.e., the compulsive need to continue taking the drug. Various writers (2, 3, 23, 37) have emphasized that despite the traditional preoccupation with physical dependence, the most important influence on the behavior of the drug user is psychological dependence. The term is merely a descriptive name, and the dynamics of the phenomenon can best be explained in terms of theories arising from experimental psychology. According to this theory a subject who is disturbed by a stimulus of some kind can make many possible responses to it. If one response is followed closely enough by correction of the disturbance, i.e., a reward, then that response is said to be reinforced so that the next time the stimulus occurs the subject is more likely to make that response than any other. In the case of drug-taking behavior the nature of the stimulus and of the reward depends upon the personality of the user and on the pharmacological effects of the drug. The strength of reinforcement depends on the temporal relation between the taking of the drug and the onset, as well as intensity, of its subjectively perceived effects. Therefore, this is markedly influenced by the dose and manner of administration.

The primary central effect of amphetamine is stimulation of the arousal system by a mechanism which has not yet been fully elucidated, but probably involving adrenergic receptors in the reticular activating system (7). The observable effects of this stimulation are increased sensory acuity, as shown by the studies of Turner (43) on olfaction and of Besser (5) on flicker fusion, shortened reaction times, faster learning, faster flow of ideas and associations, and postponement of fatigue (10, 22). These effects are likely to be perceived as pleasurable by individuals who see themselves as inadequate, and the sense of power and mastery conferred by the drug may give rise to exhilaration or euphoria. Stein and his collaborators (41) have proposed a more direct mechanism of euphoria based on the idea that amphetamine and other stimulants directly sensitize those structures in the brain which have been called the reward system. This is a set of connected neuronal structures which animals will voluntarily stimulate via implanted electrodes, even in preference to taking food or water, or the avoidance of pain. This system, therefore, has been suggested as a possible mediator of pleasurable or rewarding sensation. Consistent with this idea, recent experimental studies in animals (36) have shown that amphetamine has primary reinforcing properties. Against this view is the fact that the very same actions of amphetamine, involving heightened arousal and closer contact with the environment, may be perceived as unpleasurable or frightening by those who prefer to evade or withdraw from external reality.

Popular lore attributes a particularly strong euphoriant action to methamphetamine. Experimental evidence does not support this belief since many investigators find the central actions of amphetamine and methamphetamine indistinguishable (10, 32). Methamphetamine and *d*-amphetamine are very similar in potency and about twice as potent as racemic amphetamine. Methamphetamine does have a higher lipid solubility than amphetamine (44), and, at least in theory, it should therefore have a more rapid onset of action. However, clinical observation has shown that even experienced users may be unable to distinguish between the effects of cocaine and methamphetamine (26) when taken intravenously. Indeed in Sweden the most popular stimulant drug used in this way has been phenmetrazine (2, p. 220). Furthermore, in Toronto, Marshman and Gibbins (31) have found that nearly 40 per cent of street samples alleged to be "speed" consist of drugs other than methamphetamine. These include *d*-amphetamine, ephedrine, MDA,* and caffeine (30). This suggests that the perceived effects are largely common to the whole group of psychomotor stimulants. The expressed preference for methamphetamine may therefore reflect mainly the fact that it was originally the most readily available injectable preparation.

The strength of reinforcement, therefore, and hence the degree of the resulting dependence, are based upon the amount of drug and the manner in which it is taken. There is a tendency in the current North American literature to draw a sharp distinction between low-dose oral use and high-dose intravenous use of amphetamines. In fact this distinction is not as sharp as is frequently implied. First, the earlier literature (22) contains many well-documented case histories of users who consumed very large doses orally, as much as one gram or more daily. Second, many published accounts of intravenous use are vague about specific doses, and Kramer *et al.* (26) have pointed out that the average dose taken by the regular user is 100–300 mg, a dose quite comparable to those taken orally in many cases of amphetamine dependence (22). Third, the size of the doses taken by "speed" users cannot be accepted at face value. In Toronto for example, Tookey (42) states that street samples of "speed" are only about 25 per cent methamphetamine and 75 per cent inert diluents. Gibbins (17), in weighing "street grams," found them to range from 60 to 100 mg, with an average weight of 80 mg. The actual doses

*MDA = 3,4-methylenedioxyamphetamine.

TABLE XIV

OBSERVATIONS BY R. J. GIBBINS ON INTRAVENOUS DOSES OF AMPHETAMINE USED BY MEMBERS OF A TORONTO "SPEED" COMMUNITY

Case	Sex	Age	Samples, examined	Average single dose* (mg)	Frequency per 24 hours	Total daily dose* (mg)	Body weight (kg)	Total daily dose (mg/kg)	Duration of use (years)	Other drugs used
1	M	24	5	225	2	450	62.2	6.6	6	Minor tranquilizers, barbiturates, cannabis, alcohol, LSD
2	M	20	3	425	2-3	850-1275	72.7	11.7-17.5	5	Cannabis, minor tranquilizers, barbiturates
3	M	18	2	225	5-6	1125-1350	65.9	17.0-20.5	2	Barbiturates, minor tranquilizers, cannabis, alcohol
4	F	18	3	475	3	1425	56.8	25.0	1	Barbiturates, minor tranquilizers, cannabis
5	F	17	3	50	1	50	59.0	0.8	1	Cannabis
6	M	17	3	240	5-6	1200-1440	52.3	22.9-27.5	1	Barbiturates, minor tranquilizers, cannabis, heroin
7	F	18	3	400	3	1200	53.2	22.5	1.5	Barbiturates, minor tranquilizers
8	M	22	2	300	5	1500	63.6	23.6	5	Heroin, barbiturates
9	F	18	3	275	5-6	1375-1650	56.8	24.2-29.0	1.5	Cannabis, minor tranquilizers
10	F	18	3	325	6-8	1950-2600	68.2	28.6-38.1	2	?
11	F	18	3	300	2-3	600-900	45.4	13.2-19.8	2	?
12	M	20	3	245	3-4	735-980	75.0	9.9-13.0	3	Minor tranquilizers, alcohol
13	M	17	3	185	2-3	370-555	68.2	5.4-8.1	1.5	?
14	F	17	3	275	3-4	825-1000	59.1	13.9-18.6	1.5	Cannabis

*Figures shown represent gross weight. Chemical analysis indicated that methamphetamine constituted as little as 50 per cent of the weight of many of the samples.

therefore may not be nearly as large as they are claimed to be. Gibbins has kindly made available to us observations gathered by him during an extended study of a Toronto "speed" community. His descriptions of the social functioning of the group will be published elsewhere, but Table XIV contains data on the doses taken by members of the group. To our knowledge, his is the only study in which illicit samples have been systematically examined. The striking feature is that the daily dosage is not much greater than the larger doses shown in Table VIII of this monograph (pp. 42–7). Though the average dose in the "speed" group is clearly larger, there is evident overlap of the ranges. Moreover, analysis of the samples obtained by Gibbins indicated that as little as 50 per cent of the actual weight consisted of methamphetamine (30).

The most important feature, therefore, appears to be the use of the intravenous route. It is a clear maxim of behavioral analysis that the shorter the time that elapses between the making of a response and the delivery of the reinforcer (in this case the perceived drug effect), the stronger is the reinforcement. Intravenous injection is an excellent example because the desired effects are felt within seconds of the injection rather than the half an hour or more required after oral intake. It is therefore not surprising that the pattern of intravenous use rapidly becomes more intense, compulsive, and all-absorbing. One consequence is that the frequency of injection increases, so that the user may sustain an amphetamine binge with practically no sleep for several days, until he is forced by fatigue to terminate it. In contrast the oral user can maintain a less intense pace for many months on end.

Another consequence of intravenous injection is the development of the "needle freak." Many stimuli which are not in themselves reinforcing can acquire reinforcing properties by being paired with effective reinforcers. For example, the click of the lever which a rat must press in order to obtain a food reward becomes, by its association with the food, a partial reward in itself. In a comparable manner the act of injection, through its close association with the subsequent drug effect, may in itself become rewarding (15).* Users report positive effects even before the needle is removed from the vein, yet our knowledge of circulatory

*A striking example of this phenomenon was noted many years ago, in experiments involving repeated injection of cocaine in a dog (41a).

physiology makes it impossible to believe that the drug could have produced an effect in the brain within that time. It is even possible that the alleged preference for impure clandestinely made methamphetamine rather than commercially prepared drug may be due to the local irritant effects of impurities which would act as an immediate partial reinforcer. The bizarre reports (42) of intravenous injections of pharmacologically inert materials are testimony to the importance of the act of injection in the development of patterns of dependence.

There are at least four important implications of this fact for the subsequent history of the drug user. First, the strength of reinforcement associated with intravenous injection of amphetamine is so great that the dependence is extremely difficult to overcome by treatment. Relapses are the rule, and the prognosis is at least as bad as in opiate dependence. The second implication, an approach to therapy which merits consideration, stems directly from the principles of behavior therapy. If a central consideration is the intravenous route of administration, then conditioned avoidance therapy aimed specifically at creating an aversion to injections might be a useful adjunct to other therapies. Third, as the injection itself becomes a significant part of the total reinforcement, there is a tendency for the user to become needle-dependent. The possibility must be considered that such users are more likely to try injection of a variety of drugs, including opiates, because the specific drug effects may become secondary to rapid reinforcement by intravenous injection of almost any active substance. Fourth, the use of the intravenous route introduces a number of secondary hazards not encountered with oral use. The transmission of viral hepatitis by unsterile needles is an example (12). Another is the production of multiple microembolism by injection of particulate material such as aqueous suspensions of cannabis (21, 25). Phlebitis, abscesses, septicemia, and bacterial endocarditis are among the well-known complications (22). Another complication in "speed" users which has recently attracted considerable attention is the occurrence of necrotizing angiitis which may give rise to multiple microaneurysms or hemorrhages in various organs (9, 29).

It is not the purpose of this appendix to review in detail

156

all the problems associated with amphetamine dependence. Amphetamine toxicity has been reviewed in this monograph, and other reviews in depth are those of Ellinwood (14) on amphetamine psychosis, of Brill and Hirose (8) on public health aspects, and of Cox and Smart (11) on clinical and epidemiological features. It has been our purpose here, by calling attention to certain fundamental principles of psychopharmacology, to put in perspective the relative importance of the various factors contributing to the production of amphetamine dependence.

References

1. ALLES, C. A.: The comparative physiological actions of *dl*-β-phenylisopropylamines, J. Pharmacol. & Exper. Therap., **47**: 339–54, 1933.
2. BEJEROT, N.: Addiction and Society, p. 24. Springfield, Charles C Thomas, 1970.
3. BELL, D. S.: Addiction to stimulants, M.J. Australia, **i**: 41–5, 1967.
4. BENAKIS, A., & THOMASSET, M.: Metabolism of amphetamines and their interaction with other drugs. In: Abuse of Central Stimulants, ed. by F. Sjoqvist and M. Tottie, pp. 409–35. New York, Raven Press, 1969.
5. BESSER, C. M.: Centrally acting drugs and auditory flutter. In: Drugs and Sensory Functions, ed. by A. Herxheimer, pp. 199–206. London, J. & A. Churchill Ltd., 1968.
6. BEWLEY, T. H.: Recent changes in the pattern of drug abuse in London and the United Kingdom. In: The Pharmacological and Epidemiological Aspects of Adolescent Drug Dependence, ed. by C. W. M. Wilson, pp. 197–220. Toronto, Pergamon Press, 1968.
7. BRADLEY, P. B., & KEY, B. J.: The effect of drugs on the arousal responses produced by electrical stimulation of the reticular formation of the brain, Electroenceph. Clin. Neurophysiol., **10**: 97–110, 1958.
8. BRILL, H., & HIROSE, T.: The rise and fall of a methamphetamine epidemic: Japan 1945–55, Seminars Psychiat., **1**: 179–92, 1969.
9. CITRON, B. P., HALPERN, M., MCCARRON, M., LUNDBERG, G. D., MCCORMICK, R., PINCUS, I. J., TATTER, D., & HAVERBACK, B. J.: Necrotizing angiitis associated with drug abuse, New England J. Med., **283**: 1003–11, 1970.
10. COLE, S. O.: Experimental effects of amphetamine: A review, Psychol. Bull., **68**: 81–90, 1967.
11. COX, C., & SMART, R. G.: The nature and extent of speed use in North America, Canad. M.A.J., **102**: 724–9, 1970.
12. DAVIS, L. E., KALOUSEK, G., & RUBENSTEIN, E.: Hepatitis associated with illicit use of intravenous methamphetamine, Pub. Health Rep., **85**: 809–13, 1970.
13. EDELEANO, L.: Ueber einige Derivate der Phenylmethacrylsäure und der Phenylisobuttersäure, Berichte Deut. Chem. Ges., **20**: 616–22, 1887.
14. ELLINWOOD, E. H., Jr.: Amphetamine psychosis: a multidimensional process, Seminars Psychiat., **1**: 208–26, 1969.
15. ELLINWOOD, E. H., Jr.: "Accidental conditioning" with chronic methamphetamine intoxication: implications for a theory of drug habituation, Psychopharmacologia (Berlin), **21**: 131–8, 1971.
16. ELLISON, T., SIEGEL, M., SILVERMAN, A. G., & OKUN, R.: Comparative metabolism of *dl*-3H-amphetamine hydrochloride in tolerant and non-tolerant cats, Proc. West Pharmacol. Soc., **1**: 75–7, 1968.

17. GIBBINS, R. J.: Personal communication.
18. GIBBINS, R. J., KALANT, H., LeBLANC, A. E., & CLARK, J. W.: The effects of chronic administration of ethanol on startle thresholds in rats, Psychopharmacologia (Berlin), **19**: 95–104, 1971.
19. GOLDBERG, L.: Drug abuse in Sweden, Bull. Narcot., **20**(1): 1–31 & (2), 9–36, 1968.
20. GRIFFITH, J.: A study of illicit amphetamine drug traffic in Oklahoma City, Am. J. Psychiat., **123**: 560–9, 1966.
21. HENDERSON, A. H., & PUGSLEY, D. J.: Collapse after intravenous use of hashish, Brit. M.J., **3**: 229–30, 1968.
22. KALANT, O. J.: The Amphetamines: Toxicity and Addiction. Toronto, University of Toronto Press, 1966.
23. KALANT, H., & KALANT, O. J.: Drugs, Society and Personal Choice, p. 76. Don Mills, Ont., General Publishing, 1971.
24. KALES, J. D.: Addiction and drug-induced sleep alterations, Ann. Intern. Med., **70**: 602–5, 1969.
25. KING, A. B., & COWEN, D. L.: Effect of intravenous injection of marihuana, J.A.M.A., **210**: 724-5, 1969.
26. KRAMER, J. C., FISCHMAN, V. S., & LITTLEFIELD, D. C.: Amphetamine abuse: pattern and effects of high doses taken intravenously, J.A.M.A., **201**: 305–9, 1967.
27. LEAKE, C. D.: The Amphetamines—Their Actions and Uses. Springfield, Charles C Thomas, 1958.
28. LeBLANC, A. E.: Unpublished observations.
29. MARGOLIS, M. T., & NEWTON, T. H.: Methamphetamine ("speed") arteritis, Neuroradiology, **2**: 179–82, 1971.
30. MARSHMAN, J. A.: Unpublished observations.
31. MARSHMAN, J. A., & GIBBINS, R. J.: A note on the composition of illicit drugs, Ont. Med. Rev., Sept. 1970, pp. 1–3.
32. MARTIN, W. R., SLOAN, J. W., SAPIRA, J. D., & JASINSKI, D. R.: Physiologic, subjective, and behavioral effects of amphetamine, methamphetamine, ephedrine, phenmetrazine, and methylphenidate in man, Clin. Pharmacol. Therap., **12**: 245–58, 1971.
33. MASAKI, T.: The amphetamine problem in Japan, W.H.O. Techn. Rep. Ser., **102**: 14–21, 1956.
34. OSWALD, I., & THACORE, V. R.: Amphetamine and phenmetrazine addiction: physiological abnormalities in the abstinence syndrome, Brit. M.J., **2**: 427–31, 1963.
35. SANO, I., & NAGASAKA: Ueber chronische Weckaminsucht in Japan, Fortschr. Neurol. Psychiat., **24**: 391–4, 1956.
36. SCHUSTER, C. R., & THOMPSON, T.: Self administration of and behavioral dependence on drugs, Ann. Rev. Pharmacol., **9**: 483–502, 1969.
37. SEEVERS, M. H.: Psychopharmacological elements of drug dependence, J.A.M.A., **206**: 1263–6, 1968.
38. SIEGEL, M., ELLISON, T., SILVERMAN, A. G., & OKUN, R.: Tissue distribution of dl-3H-amphetamine HCl in tolerant and non-tolerant cats, Proc. West. Pharmacol. Soc., **1**: 90–4, 1968.
39. SMITH, D. E.: Physical vs. psychological dependence and tolerance in high-dose methamphetamine abuse, Clin. Toxicol., **2**: 99–103, 1969.
40. SMITH, R. C.: The world of the Haight Ashbury speed freak, J. Psychedelic Drugs, **2**: 172–88, 1969.
41. STEIN, L., & WISE, C. D.: Behavioral pharmacology of central stimulants. In: Principles of Psychopharmacology, ed. by W. G. Clark and J. del Giudice, pp. 313–25. New York, Academic Press Inc., 1970.

158

41a. TATUM, A. L., & SEEVERS, M. H.: Experimental cocaine addiction, J. Pharmacol. & Exper. Therap., **36**: 401–10, 1929.
42. TOOKEY, H.: The increasing use of methamphetamine ("speed") among young people. Unpublished manuscript.
43. TURNER, P.: Amphetamines and smell threshold in man. In: Drugs and Sensory Functions, ed. by A. Herxheimer, pp. 91–97. London, J. & A. Churchill Ltd., 1968.
44. VREE, T. B., & VAN ROSSUM, J. M.: Kinetics of metabolism and excretion of amphetamines in man. In: International Symposium on Amphetamines and Related Compounds, ed. by E. Costa and S. Garattini, pp. 165–90. New York, Raven Press, 1970.
45. WORLD HEALTH ORGANIZATION, Expert Committee on Addiction-Producing Drugs: 13th Report, W.H.O. Techn. Rep. Ser., **273**: 14–15, 1964.

C. The Nature and Extent of Speed Use in North America*

CAROLE COX and REGINALD G. SMART

IN 1965 the World Health Organization stated its concern over the epidemic-like spread of amphetamine abuse (speed), particularly among young people in certain countries (24). The increasing use of the amphetamines has been referred to in other literature (15, 18) and is a cause of growing concern to the general public and the health-care professions.

Speed is the street name for methamphetamine hydrochloride (Methedrine) when it is injected intravenously. Methedrine is made of a powder-like raw material known as crystals. It is usually sold in capsules and then mixed with water for injection (10).

Several important social and health problems are created by speed use. The use of common needles presents the dangers of serum hepatitis as illustrated in cases presented by Johnson (13). Unwin (23) has also referred to the increasing high rate of serum hepatitis in hippie communities and its relationship to speed. The second set of problems concerns the toxic, addictive, and dependency-producing effects of speed and the social and psychological disturbances created by heavy speed use.

An example of the problems involved is the methamphetamine epidemic that occurred in Japan between 1945 and 1955, at a time when both the United States and Japanese military organizations dumped their surplus amphetamines into the Japanese market. The drugs were available without prescription and soon became very popular. At its peak this epidemic affected about 2,000,000

*This paper was published originally in the *Canadian Medical Association Journal*, vol. 102 (1970), pp. 724–9.

160

persons, mostly young men. It was finally controlled through strict government legislation and extensive public education (4). The numbers of speed users in North America have probably not reached this level, although only rough estimates are available for any particular city.

As this is a relatively new drug problem in North America, there is little information available on the causes and effects of current speed use. Although it is certainly relevant, much of the literature on amphetamines deals only with low-dosage use and not with high-dose intravenous administration. The present paper is a review of the literature pertaining to the nature and extent of speed use in North America. An attempt will be made to discuss the effects of speed as well as the backgrounds and characteristics of its users.

The Acute Effects of Speed

One of the attractions of speed is the swiftness of its effects. Its full impact can be felt before the needle is removed from the arm (5). A very sharp awakening is felt as the drug rushes through the blood stream; this rush has been compared to an electric shock or to being splashed in the face with ice water (5). This initial feeling is also said to be one of intense pleasure analogous to a complete body orgasm (15, 20). For some users the immediate pleasure from the injection is a prime reason for using speed; any later effect of the drug is of only secondary consequence (19).

As the speed circulates through the blood stream certain immediate physiological changes occur: the blood pressure is raised, the pulse rate is increased, the pupils dilate and vision is blurred, and there is a loss of appetite (7). Other pharmacological effects are constriction of blood vessels with blanching of mucous membranes, variability in cardiac output, dilation of the bronchi, relaxation of the intestinal muscle, and increased blood sugar, blood coagulability, and muscle tension(16).

The physiological symptoms that are commonly noted are insomnia, lack of appetite, difficulties in micturition, thirst, diaphoresis, and increased energy (8). These symptoms are accompanied by certain behavioral states which include heightened activity and alertness and a feeling of euphoria (7).

161

Amphetamines act as general stimulants of the central nervous system. Subjectively this stimulation is felt as a sense of increased energy and self-confidence, faster and more efficient thought and decision-making, and a feeling of well-being (14). However, as tolerance to the drug develops, the dose is raised and the frequency of the injections increased (15). The sense of cleverness, self-confidence, and clearer thinking which are experienced at smaller doses becomes marred by rapid mood changes and often frightening illusions and hallucinations (15). Concentration on any one idea becomes difficult as thoughts go racing through the head. Carey and Mandel (5), in their study of speed users in California, observed that after heavy doses users could not sit still and were also incapable of doing heavy tasks; pure quietness or stillness is practically unknown in speed scenes.

At times the world may actually get out of control; it is then that a "freakout" occurs. The hyperactivity resulting from the increased energy may lead to aggressive behavior, while a preoccupation with one's own thoughts and actions can develop into compulsive, meaningless behavior, such as the stringing of beads for hours (5).

Large doses of amphetamines make the user want to interact socially, but his ability to do so in a rational manner becomes severely limited. Paranoid reactions may develop and make the users extremely suspicious of their friends and very difficult to get along with. Carey and Mandel (5) have observed violence which resulted from presumed insults. On the other hand, Kramer, Fischman, and Littlefield (15), from their interviews with 36 amphetamine abusers at the California Rehabilitation Center, found the paranoid symptoms were often regarded humorously when their occurrence became expected.

Because of their desire for sociability and because few people can tolerate them, speed users tend to come together. Rawlin (17) has described how speed users in a midwestern city would congregate at a "splash" house. These houses are often owned by pushers, so that drugs can be bought there and the company of other users enjoyed. Carey and Mandel (5) have described the "flash" houses in the San Francisco area where users congregate to shoot speed. These houses are also often owned by pushers, but sometimes they are owned by the users themselves. Particular houses become very

162

popular and very crowded as their reputation grows. They tend to be rather impermanent owing to violent behavior on the part of the residents, fear of the police, and failure to pay rents.

Amphetamines have been reported to create or enhance sexual pleasure, although there is some disagreement as to the frequency of these effects. After speed use, ejaculation and female orgasm may be delayed so that sexual activity may continue for hours (15). When orgasm finally occurs it has been described as being far more pleasurable than without the drug. Many of Kramer's subjects stated that their primary reason for taking amphetamines was for its effect on their sexual powers. On the other hand, Bell (2) claims that only about one-third of the users actually report an increase in sexuality, and that the sexually inhibited may actually become more so.

The "run" (period during which speed is continuously injected) is finally terminated for a variety of reasons. There may be exhaustion, frightening hallucinations, or an inability to get further supplies (19). The crash, the coming down from the drug, may actually be very severe in that there may be strong anxiety reactions and depression, extreme irritability, or even violent behavior or suicide. The crasher has an overpowering desire to sleep and may do so for several days; upon arousal he has a voracious appetite. He may also awake with an extreme depression, and to escape from this he may begin to shoot speed again, thus beginning another cycle.

The Chronic Effects of Speed

The chronic effects of speed have been widely publicized in the statement "speed kills," but this succinctly summarizes an assumption and not a proven fact. To date there is no evidence to support the belief that speed users have a shortened life span or that speed use, in itself, is fatal. Currently there is very little scientific information concerning many of the presumed effects of the chronic use of speed.

It has still not been decided whether the continual regular use of speed actually leads to physical addiction. Kalant (14) claims that, according to the definition given by the World Health Organization in 1957, addiction to amphetamines does exist. Physical dependence in chronic abusers has been indicated by the discovery of certain abnormal electroencephalographic and electro-occulographic patterns which occur during withdrawal but end when the amphetamine is restored. These patterns and the tolerance which develops led Kalant (14) to conclude that addiction does develop. The slow elimination of the drug from the body may make it difficult to detect severe withdrawal symptoms.

Smith (18) believes that withdrawal symptoms can occur in heavy speed users and that they may parallel those seen in narcotics addicts. After many continuous "runs" he has noticed severe gastrointestinal cramps as well as heavy lethargy and sleepiness in the users. These symptoms lead him to believe in the existence of withdrawal symptoms and that the possibility and nature of physical dependence should be investigated.

The regular and prolonged use of speed appears to have definite psychological effects. Carey and Mandel (5) state that after many months of continuous use the users' brains "get scrambled"; they are unable to make mental connections, their memory becomes impaired, and, particularly, there is an inability to remember very recent events. The study by Kramer, Fischman, and Littlefield (15) supports these findings, since one-third of their 36 users had impairment of memory and concentration although no tests were performed to determine whether temporary or permanent brain damage had occurred.

A similar uncertainty exists about the nature and frequency of amphetamine psychoses. Kalant (14) reviewed 210 cases and concluded that the psychosis is the most serious and frequently reported toxic effect of chronic amphetamine consumption. Yet it is still not known what proportion of heavy users actually develop psychoses or what events may precipitate them.

Ellinwood (9) has suggested that the development of the psychosis depends on the interaction of a predisposed personality, the environment, and the stimulation of the central nervous system arousal system. He believes that psychopathic and schizophrenic individuals are more prone to abuse amphetamines than other diagnostic groups, and that schizophrenics and borderline schizophrenics are most susceptible to the development of psychoses. Ellinwood based his theory on his work with amphetamine abusers

164

in the Narcotics Hospital at Lexington, Kentucky. Hekimian and Gershon (12) found that the condition of 41 per cent of the amphetamine abusers admitted to the Bellevue Psychiatric Hospital could be diagnosed as schizophrenia before they had started taking the drug. The pre-addiction diagnoses were made after admission to the hospital for treatment by means of the patients' own descriptions of their pre-drug personalities; the reliability of these diagnoses may therefore be rather limited.

The amphetamine psychosis itself has been described by Connell (6) as a paranoid psychosis in a setting of clear consciousness; it is easily mistaken for paranoid schizophrenia. Distinguishing features of the amphetamine psychoses are highly developed and fixed delusions, repetitious compulsive behavior, and the ability to remember clearly events occurring during the psychotic episode (9). The psychosis is usually of short duration and disappears within a week or less after withdrawal from the drug. This adds to the difficulty of studying such psychoses, as many probably develop and disappear without being seen by a physician.

The paranoid state is almost past by the time the user awakens from the exhaustive state following a run (15). Although Smith (19) has observed a prolonged hallucinosis in which auditory and visual hallucinations persisted for weeks after the acute reaction had ended, such an effect is not common and it is not known whether the drug or personality factors are mainly responsible. Smith (18) found that the psychotics were extremely difficult to treat, that they often required hospitalization, and that many patients developed an acute anxiety reaction after a long speed binge had ended. In this state the individual is usually nervous, anxious, and agitated but is easily helped by a supportive environment.

Smith (18) has also stated that amphetamines often lead to paranoid reactions after prolonged use. The element of prolonged use is also mentioned by Kalant (14) and Ellinwood (8) as being important to the development of psychoses. Kramer and his colleagues (15) have stated that paranoid symptoms seldom occur during oral use or even after the first few months of intravenous use and that they develop after a long period of continual use.

The psychosis is believed to intensify as a "run" continues,

165

usually developing around the second or third day, the hallucinations becoming progressively more bizarre as the run continues (9, 15). Kramer and his associates (15) have stated that, in their cases, paranoid symptoms were expected and were not taken too seriously, although during a long run it became more difficult to accept the delusions as being unreal. Paranoid beliefs were often related to the user's own law violations, individuals believing they were being watched by the police or becoming suspicious of their friends. Ellinwood (8) found that those patients who were paranoid before taking amphetamines had the more common delusions of being persecuted by Martians, evil spirits, and communists.

In contrast to the high proportion of schizophrenic reactions reported in the West, the Japanese amphetamine episode showed a wider variety of psychiatric symptoms. Brill and Hirose (4) report that Tatetsu found 8 per cent tending to be psychopathic, 19 per cent mixed manic and schizophrenic, 23 per cent manic-depressive, and 31 per cent in apathetic exhausted states. Tatetsu also states that as police surveillance became more severe the psychoses tended to reflect more anxiety about the police and projection mechanisms developed. This may be the parallel of the paranoid states seen in western psychoses, where the form of the psychotic beliefs is often related to legal violations.

As well as causing abnormal psychological states, continual speed use may bring about certain physical conditions. These include hepatitis, malnutrition, skin abscesses, and other dermatological problems (20). Smith (18) has stated that speed may produce a direct toxic effect on the liver, since he has seen many cases of hepatitis which appear to differ from serum hepatitis. He has also observed many cases of acute abdominal pain resembling appendicitis and many respiratory problems. However, no fatalities resulting from any of these medical conditions have been reported.

There is no information available on mortality rates among speed users, and it is not certain that speed itself is a lethal drug. Kalant (14) has cited examples of people who have used amphetamines for long periods of time, up to 16 years, in large doses, with no signs of physical or mental toxic effects or addiction. On the other hand, she has reported instances where death has occurred after doses taken on medical prescription. This, she believes, indicates the wide variability in individual response. Regular users of speed have been known to inject 15,000 mg in one day (15). Such high doses could be lethal if tolerance through continuous use had not been built up (7). From those who mention (5, 9, 10, 15, 20) the high doses which regular users tolerate, there is no statement of mortality rates among regular users in whom tolerance has developed.

Smith's experiments on white mice show the group toxicity of amphetamines* (19). The LD-50 for *d*-amphetamine proved to be 100 mg per kg when an animal was kept isolated, but when the animals were placed in groups of eight the LD-50 decreased to 25 mg per kg; thus, the association of the animals increased the toxicity of the drug four times. At 25 mg the mice were hyperexcitable and aggressive and attempted to kill each other, but with higher dosages they became progressively more disorganized and unable to attack.

Smith has related this group toxicity factor to the violent and hyperexcitable states often seen in speed users in group settings. He claims that an immediate cause of the increase in violence in the Haight-Ashbury area of San Francisco was the increasing use of amphetamines and their group-toxic response. Perhaps, in this indirect way, speed may kill.

The Extent of Speed Use

In 1958 the production of amphetamines in the United States was about 75,000 pounds or 3.5 billion tablets, enough to provide 20 tablets for every person in the country (14). Amphetamines are not produced in Canada but are imported in bulk either in powder or as finished products by licensed dealers. In 1962 imports amounted to 424 kg, which would be enough to provide every man, woman, and child with 4.5 tablets for the year (14). It is believed that amphetamine consumption is lower in Canada than in the United States, but there is no recent evidence regarding the actual consumption or the amount available on the black market.

Amphetamines have been widely prescribed by physicians for

*Group toxicity refers to mortality when animals are housed in cages with other similarly treated animals.

the treatment of narcolepsy, depression, and obesity. Their misuse has resulted when patients have begun taking them primarily for their side effects. Smith (18) has described the "housewife syndrome" in which women take prescribed diet pills three or four times a day, not for diet control but for euphoria or mood elevation. It is very unlikely that these women will become speed freaks; their environment and their needs are such as would not allow them to join the speed world. Griffith (11), in his study of amphetamine abuse in Oklahoma City, found that women for whom the drug was prescribed for weight control or emotional problems had not been told that it could become habit-forming; none of the women seeking help from physicians for amphetamine dependence had any prior knowledge of the fact that they could become dependent on the drug.

The use of amphetamines is very popular among college youths and teenagers. Rawlin (17) states that during the late forties to the late fifties amphetamines became part of the final exam ritual when students used the drug to help them cram all night. He believes that this pattern laid the foundation for later abuse. Smith and Blachly (21), in their study of amphetamine use among medical students at the University of Oregon, found that just under half of the students had used amphetamines, and the majority of the users had used them more than once. Seven per cent of the users had taken doses of 30 to 100 mg, thus exceeding the normal therapeutic dose of 5 to 12 mg a day. One of the users started taking the drug intravenously in doses of 125 to 200 mg a day. There is actually little information available as to how many college students progress from oral amphetamine use to high-dose intravenous use.

High-school students also appear to be showing an increasing rate of amphetamine use. Smith (18) found that 22 per cent of the 11th and 12th graders in a San Francisco high school had taken amphetamines orally once or twice, and 75 per cent of the users had taken them three or more times. Blum et al. (3) found that 13 per cent of the students in a suburban San Francisco high school had used stimulants. The use of these drugs is not confined to the west coast of the United States. In a study of Toronto high-school students (1), it was shown that 7.3 per cent of all students between grades 7 and 13 had used some sort of stimulant in the previous six-month period. These studies are limited in that they do not differentiate between amphetamines taken as prescriptions and those taken illicitly; nor do they differentiate between oral amphetamines and speed.

In one study which provides information directly about speed use in London, Ontario (22), 5 per cent of the students admitted they had actually taken speed. More studies of this type, which specifically refer to speed as distinct from stimulants, are needed.

Although it is widely believed that the number of speed users is growing, there is little reliable information to support or negate this belief. During the summer of 1967, 310 cases of amphetamine abuse were seen in the medical clinic in the Haight-Ashbury area of San Francisco. Throughout the year the clinic continued to see three to five amphetamine-related problems a day (18). Smith has stated that speed has become the major drug problem in Haight-Ashbury. Figures on the number of speed users being seen by other clinics and in other cities are not available and hence it is difficult to determine reliably even the number of speed abusers.

Personality Characteristics and Social Backgrounds of Speed Users

Only a few systematic studies of the backgrounds of speed users have been made. None of these contains a sample larger than 36, and all are from the San Francisco area. Nevertheless, a few generalizations about the social characteristics of speed users can be made.

Speed is attractive mainly to young people in their teens and early twenties. The amphetamine epidemic in post-war Japan involved mainly young men between the ages of 16 and 25 from the lower social classes (4). Hekimian and Gershon's (12) sample of amphetamine abusers admitted to Bellevue Psychiatric Hospital had a mean age of 24.8 years. Other studies (5, 7, 17, 18) also refer to its popularity with young people. The effects of speed appear to correspond with a youthful desire for action, energy, and "go."

In their study of 36 amphetamine users in the California Rehabilitation Center, Kramer and his colleagues (15) differentiated the "preferential" from the "facultative" speed users. The latter prefers to take opiates, but because they are too expensive or unobtainable he takes speed instead. The preferential user takes speed because he seeks the effects which it alone produces. Almost all users of both types have experimented with other drugs, including marihuana, opiates, barbiturates, and psychedelics. Many continue to take these drugs while on speed. The speed users reported on by Fischman (10) frequently combined barbiturates or, preferably, opiates with the stimulants in order to control depression and paranoid behavior.

From their observations of the hippie community of San Francisco Davis and Munoz (7) distinguished the "heads" from the "freaks." The heads are those who primarily use LSD and other mind-expanding drugs to provide greater intellectual awareness and self-insight. They are often the spokesmen of the hippie communities, and this group includes writers, artists, and graduate students. They are likely to be in their mid- to late twenties and to be engaged in some sort of vocation. In contrast to the "heads," "freaks" are not concerned with gaining new insight or deeper understanding; they are interested in action and kicks and therefore prefer speed. The freaks include many members of motorcycle gangs.

In regard to backgrounds, it is the impression of Davis and Munoz (7) that the heads are more often from middle-class homes, whereas the freaks are more likely to come from working-class homes, although this distinction does not appear to be clearly established. LSD and speed are representative of the differences in these backgrounds. LSD symbolizes the middle-class value of self-improvement, whereas speed is symbolic of the working-class culture in its release of aggression and body stimulation. Nevertheless, distinctions between the heads and the freaks are blurred, as there are many people who shift back and forth between drugs or take whatever is available.

In their observations of the San Francisco Bay area speed scene, Carey and Mandel (5) found that most users were jobless, young, living away from home, and without any on-going reputation. Smith (18) has divided the users in the Haight-Ashbury area into three groups: sociopathic groups including motorcycle gangs, criminals, black militants; pre-psychotics, those unable to function in society; teeny-boppers, young teenagers who begin using speed

170

because it is the first drug which they encounter. The sample of speed users reported on by Kramer, Fischman, and Littlefield (15) included hippies, middle-class neurotics, former heroin addicts, and members of motorcycle gangs.

Though these studies of the characteristics and backgrounds of speed users are interesting, they are limited, in that all describe individuals from the San Francisco area, and most are concerned with only one community composed predominantly of hippies. Studies in other communities are needed.

Those inhabiting the speed world are so totally engrossed in it that any other activity is difficult to maintain. With the speed binge lasting for 36 to 72 hours and the crash lasting for several days, the user is incapacitated for a week or more. This makes it extremely difficult to maintain a steady job. Rawlin (17) claims that many users support their drug habit through petty theft or breaking into cars. Bell (2) states that shoplifting, thieving, breaking and entering are common offences committed in order to get money.

Studies have compared the personality characteristics of amphetamine users with those of heroin addicts. Ellinwood (8) found amphetamine users to be more withdrawn and resentful of authority, and to have a higher incidence of psychiatric hospitalizations than the usual addict. Of the 25 users whom he studied in the Lexington Hospital, 60 per cent had antisocial and schizoid personalities, a proportion much higher than in the general addict population. The amphetamine users also had a higher incidence of previous juvenile delinquencies and more admissions to reform schools.

Fischman's comparison (10) of narcotics addicts and stimulant users in the California Rehabilitation Center differs from Ellinwood's in that he found no differences in the modal psychiatric diagnosis. The two groups had the same basic personality disorders and neurotic characters. With regard to group behavior, the stimulant users participated more intensely and sincerely in the treatment program. They were also more sociable, adaptable, sensitive and insecure, verbal and intellectual, and had more insight than the narcotic addicts. Furthermore, in comparison with the narcotic users, speed users tended to be more literate, to have more education, probably higher IQs, and to come from higher socioeconomic backgrounds than the average narcotics user. Fischman's findings differ from those of Ellinwood and from other impressions of speed users, but no clear reason for this discrepancy is readily apparent.

Discussion

As the rapid growth of speed use is a recent phenomenon in North America, many areas require further investigation. Much of the literature on stimulants deals mainly with oral amphetamine abuse and does not examine the particular problems resulting from high-dose methamphetamine injections. This is an area where much speculation remains but there are few data, especially on the long-term consequences of heavy speed use. Longitudinal studies of the development of speed use have not been made, nor are there follow-up studies of speed users or abusers.

The phrase "speed kills" is widely quoted and, in fact, had its origin in the hippie community. It in itself is supposed to act as a deterrent to the use of speed, yet there is no evidence to confirm or deny that the phrase is true. It is often said that speed freaks have perhaps two to five years to live, but this has never been proved.

The development of the amphetamine psychosis is also an area where more research is needed. It is still not known what proportion of users actually develop a psychosis or how many such psychoses are misdiagnosed as schizophrenia. Whether certain personalities are predisposed to the development of the psychoses, or whether all regular users will eventually develop them, is also uncertain.

There are contrary views as to what aspects of speed use are of primary importance to the user. Is it the initial injection and the jolt which it produces, or is it the euphoric effects of speed itself? Knowing more about the reasons for its use would create a basis for understanding the motivations and characteristics of its users. Possibly a wide variety of reasons exist for its use, and these distinctions may be crucial to an understanding of the total problem.

It has been stated that the world of speed is totally engrossing and that it is difficult to maintain a life outside that world (5). To maintain a pattern of just weekend use would be difficult, as tolerance to the drug develops and increasing doses lead to at least

172

temporary incapacity. Studies should be made to see whether occasional users can maintain an identity outside the speed scene and keep from becoming completely submerged in the world of speed.

Little has been said so far about the treatment of speed users; the reason is that successful therapy has not yet been found. Terminating speed use appears to be very difficult. Smith (19) claims this is possible only when the user is removed from the speed subcultures; otherwise the temptation to begin again is too great. Similarly, Kramer and his colleagues (15) claim that the desire of amphetamine users to return to the drug after forced treatment is comparable to the desire of heroin users. Even though many speed users have been seen in clinics, there are no good estimates of the success of treatment in terminating their speed use. However, it appears that success rates in treatment are very low. Whether or not this is mainly due to the low motivation is not known. This great dependence upon the drug which develops and the impelling need which users seem to have for it should certainly be studied. It may well be that the development of reliable therapies will depend upon more exhaustive studies of the personalities, backgrounds, and physical conditions of speed users.

References

1. ADDICTION RESEARCH FOUNDATION: A Preliminary Report on the Attitudes and Behaviour of Toronto Students in Relation to Drugs. Toronto, 1969.
2. BELL, D. S.: Addiction to stimulants, M.J. Australia, i: 41–5, 1967.
3. BLUM, H., & associates: Drugs II. Students and Drugs; College and High School Observations. San Francisco, Jossey-Bass, Inc., 1969.
4. BRILL, H., & HIROSE, T.: The rise and fall of a methamphetamine epidemic: Japan 1954–55, Seminars Psychiat., 1: 179-92, 1969.
5. CAREY, J. T., & MANDEL, J.: A San Francisco Bay Area "speed" scene, J. Health Soc. Behav., 9: 164–74, 1968.
6. CONNELL, P. H.: The use and abuse of amphetamines, Practitioner, 200: 234–43, 1968.
7. DAVIS, F., & MUNOZ, L.: Heads and freaks: patterns and meanings of drug use among hippies, J. Health Soc. Behav., 9: 156–64, 1968.
8. ELLINWOOD, E. H., JR.: Amphetamine psychosis: I. Description of the individuals and process, J. Nerv. & Ment. Dis., 144: 273–83, 1967.
9. ELLINWOOD, E. H., Jr.: Amphetamine psychosis: a multidimensional process, Seminars Psychiat., 1: 208–26, 1969.
10. FISCHMAN, V. S.: Stimulant users in the California Rehabilitation Center, Int. J. Addict., 3: 113–30, 1968.
11. GRIFFITH, J. D.: Psychiatric implication of amphetamine abuse. In: Amphetamine Abuse, ed. by J. R. Russo, p. 15. Springfield, Charles C Thomas, 1968.

173

12. HEKIMIAN, L. J., & GERSHON, S.: Characteristics of drug abusers admitted to a psychiatric hospital, J.A.M.A., **205**: 125–30, 1968.
13. JOHNSON, J. S.: Serum hepatitis and illicit drug use, Rocky Mountain M. J., **65**: 43–5, 1968.
14. KALANT, O. J.: The Amphetamines: Toxicity and Addiction. Toronto: University of Toronto Press, 1966.
15. KRAMER, J. C., FISCHMAN, V. S., & LITTLEFIELD, D. C.: Amphetamine abuse: pattern and effects of high doses taken intravenously, J.A.M.A., **201**: 305–9, 1967.
16. LEAKE, C. D.: The Amphetamines—Their Actions and Uses, p. 51. Springfield, Charles C Thomas, 1968.
17. RAWLIN, J. W.: Street level abusage of amphetamines. In: Amphetamine Abuse, ed. by J. R. Russo, p. 51. Springfield, Charles C Thomas, 1968.
18. SMITH, D. E.: Speed kills: patterns of high dose methamphetamine abuse. Paper presented at discussion on Current Problems of Drug Abuse, San Francisco, 1968.
19. SMITH, D. E.: [Medical Staff Conference] Changing drug patterns in the Haight-Ashbury, Calif. Med., **110**: 151–7, 1969.
20. SMITH, D. E.: Physical vs. psychological dependence and tolerance in high-dose methamphetamine abuse, Clin. Toxicol., **2**: 99–103, 1969.
21. SMITH, S. N., & BLACHLY, P. H.: Amphetamine usage by medical students, J. Med. Educ., **41**: 167–70, 1966.
22. STENNETT, R. G., FEENSTRA, H. J., & AHARAN, C. H.: Tobacco, alcohol and drug use reported by London secondary school students: a joint project by the Addiction Research Foundation and the Board of Education for the city of London (Preliminary Report). Addiction Research Foundation, London, Ontario, 1969.
23. UNWIN, J. R.: Illicit drug use among Canadian youth, Canad. M.A.J., **98**: 402–7, 1968.
24. WORLD HEALTH ORGANIZATION, Expert Committee on Dependence-Producing Drugs: W.H.O. Techn. Rep. Ser., **312**, 1, 1965.

References

1. ABELY, P., BOBIN, P., & GEIER, S.: Toxicomanie mixte aux amphétamines et aux dérivés de l'oxazine chez de jeunes sujets, Ann. médico-psychol., **118**: 167–72, 1960.
2. ABELY, P., RONDEPIERRE, M., & GELLMAN, C.: A propos des maladies de l'appétit. Les hyperorexies féminines pathologiques et leur fréquente évolution vers la toxicomanie. Leur opposition et leurs quelques points communs avec l'anorexie. Leur thérapeutique. Ann. médico-psychol., **121**: 593–600, 1963.
3. ALLIEZ, J.: Délire amphétaminique, Encéphale, **42**: 21–6, 1953.
4. ANDERSON, E. W., & SCOTT, W. C.: Cardiovascular effects of Benzedrine, Lancet, ii: 1461–2, 1936.
5. Anonymous (annotation): Amphetamine overdosage in an athlete, Brit. M. J., ii: 590, 1960.
6. Anonymous (To-day's drugs): "Purple hearts," Brit. M. J., ii: 670, 1962.
7. Anonymous (Annotation): Amphetamine-barbiturate combinations, Brit. M. J., ii: 1456–7, 1962.
8. Anonymous (Editorial): Addiction to amphetamines, Brit. M. J., ii: 399–400, 1963.
9. Anonymous (Editorial): Pep pill menace, Brit. M. J., i: 792, 1964.
10. Anonymous (Editorial): Control of pep pills, Brit. M. J., i: 925, 1964.
11. Anonymous (Editorial): Appetite suppressants, Lancet, i: 144, 1962.
12. Anonymous (Editorial): Amphetamine and delinquency, Lancet, ii: 452, 1964.
13. APFELBERG, B.: A case of Benzedrine Sulfate poisoning, J.A.M.A., **110**: 575–6, 1938.
14. ASKEVOLD, F.: The occurrence of paranoid incidents and abstinence delirium in abuses of amphetamine, Acta psychiat. et neurol. scandinav., **34**: 145–64, 1959.
15. ATKINSON, J. B.: Factitial thyrotoxic crisis induced by dextro-amphetamine sulfate and thyroid, Ann. Int. Med., **40**: 615–18, 1954.
16. AYACHE, C.: Episode oniroïde consécutif à une injection amphétaminique thérapeutique, Maroc. méd., **39**: 555–6, 1960.
17. BACHRICH, P. R.: New drugs of addiction? (Correspondence), Brit. M. J., i: 834–5, 1964.
18. BAHNSEN, P., JACOBSEN, E., & THESLEFF, H.: The subjective effect of beta-phenylisopropylamine sulfate on normal adults, Acta med. Scandinav., **97**: 89–131, 1938.
19. BAKST, H. J.: Daily use of Benzedrine Sulfate over a period of nine years: Report of a case, U.S. Naval Med. Bull., **43**: 1228–31, 1944.
20. BARUK, H., & JOUBERT, P.: Actions thérapeutiques et dangers des amphétamines ou amines psycho-toniques, toxicomanies et délires hallucinatoires ortédriniques, Ann. médico-psychol., **111**: 305–13, 1953.
21. BEAMISH, P., & KILOH, L. G.: Psychoses due to amphetamine consumption, J. Ment. Sc., **106**: 337–43, 1960.
22. BELL, D. S., & TRETHOWAN, W. H.: Amphetamine addiction, J. Nerv. & Ment. Dis., **133**: 489–96, 1961.

23. BELL, D. S., & TRETHOWAN, W. H.: Amphetamine addiction and disturbed sexuality, Arch. Gen. Psychiat. (Chic.), 4: 74–8, 1961.
24. BERNHEIM, J., & COX, J. N.: Coup de chaleur et intoxication amphétaminique chez un sportif, Schweiz. med. Wchnschr., 90: 322–31, 1960.
25. BETHELL, M. F.: Toxic psychosis caused by Preludin, Brit. M. J., i: 30–1, 1957.
26. BETT, W. R., HOWELLS, L. H., & MACDONALD, A. D.: Amphetamine in Clinical Medicine—Actions and Uses. Edinburgh & London, E. & S. Livingston, Ltd., 1955.
27. BEYER, K. H., & SKINNER, J. T.: The detoxication and excretion of beta-phenylisopropylamine (Benzedrine), J. Pharmacol. & Exper. Therap., 68: 419–32, 1940.
28. BLOOMBERG, W.: End results of use of large doses of amphetamine sulfate over prolonged periods, New England J. Med., 222: 946–8, 1940.
29. BONHOFF, G., & LEWRENZ, H.: Ueber Weckamine (Pervitin und Benzedrin). Berlin, J. S. Springer, 1954.
30. BRANDON, S.: Addiction to amphetamines (Correspondence), Brit. M. J., ii: 1204, 1963.
31. BRANDON, S., & SMITH, D.: Amphetamines in general practice, J. Coll. Gen. Pract., 5: 603–6, 1962.
31a. BREITNER, C.: Appetite suppressing drugs as an etiologic factor in mental illness, Psychosomatics, 4: 327–33, 1963.
32. BROWN, C. T.: Benzedrine habituation, Mil. Surgeon, 104: 365–70, 1949.
33. BROWNLEE, G., & WILLIAMS, G. W.: Potentiation of amphetamine and pethidine by monoamineoxidase inhibitors, Lancet, i: 669 & 1323, 1963.
34. BURN, J. L.: Addiction to amphetamines (Correspondence), Brit. M. J., ii: 481, 1962.
35. CAPLAN, J.: Habituation to diethylpropion (Tenuate), Canad. M. A. J., 88: 943–4, 1963.
36. CARR, R. B.: Acute psychotic reaction after inhaling methylamphetamine, Brit. M. J., i: 1476, 1954.
37. CARRATALÁ, R., & CALZETTA, J. C.: Un nuevo peligro moderno: las aminas despertadoras; tentativa de suicidio con estimulex, Semana méd., ii: 985–8, 1943.
38. CHANCE, M. R. A.: Factors influencing the toxicity of sympathomimetic amines to solitary mice, J. Pharmacol. & Exper. Therap., 89: 289–96, 1947.
39. CHAPMAN, A. H.: Paranoid psychoses associated with amphetamine usage, a clinical note, Am. J. Psychiat., 111: 43–5, 1954.
40. CLEIN, L. J.: Toxic psychosis caused by Preludin, Brit. M. J., i: 282, 1957.
41. CLEIN, L. J., & BENADY, D. R.: Case of diethylpropion addiction, Brit. M. J., ii: 456, 1962.
42. CONNELL, P. H.: Amphetamine Psychosis. London, Chapman & Hall Ltd., 1958.
43. CONNELL, P. H.: Amphetamine misuse, Brit. J. Addict., 60: 9–27, 1964.
44. CORNI, L.: La tossicomania da derivati fenilpropilaminici, Riv. sper. freniat., 79: 71–100, 1955.
45. Council on Drugs (U.S.A.): Abuse of the amphetamines and pharmacologically related substances, J.A.M.A., 183: 362–3, 1963.
46. Council on Drugs (U.S.A.): The use of the terms habituation and addiction, J.A.M.A., 183: 363, 1963.
47. Council on Pharmacy and Chemistry (U.S.A.): Present status of Benzedrine Sulfate, J.A.M.A., 109: 2064–9, 1937.
48. CREMIEUX, A., CAIN, J., & RABATTU, J.: Toxicomanie alcoolique et ortédrinique chez un déséquilibré de la sexualité, Ann. médico-psychol., 106: 497–501, 1948.
49. CURRY, G. A.: Amphetamine poisoning, J.A.M.A., 140: 850, 1949.

50. DALLY, P. J.: Fatal reaction associated with tranylcypromine and methyl-amphetamine (Correspondence), Lancet, i: 1235–6, 1962.
51. DARLING, H. F.: Addiction to phenmetrazine hydrochloride, Am. J. Psychiat., 118: 558, 1961.
52. DAUBE, H.: Pervitinpsychosen, Nervenarzt, 15: 20–5, 1942.
53. DAVIES, I. J.: Benzedrine: A review of its toxic effects, with a report of a severe case of anaemia following its use, Brit. M. J., ii: 615–17, 1937.
54. DELAY, J., PICHOT, P., LEMPERIÈRE, T., & SADOUN, R.: Psychoses amphéta-miniques et pseudo-psychoses amphétaminiques, Ann. médico-psychol., 112: 51–7, 1954.
55. DEWAR, M. M., & MacCAMMOND, I.: Phenmetrazine (Correspondence), Lancet, ii: 128, 1959.
56. EHRICH, W. E., LEWY, F. H., & KRUMBHAAR, E. B.: Experimental studies upon the toxicity of Benzedrine Sulphate in various animals, Am. J. M. Sc., 198: 785–803, 1939.
57. EHRICH, W. E., & KRUMBHAAR, E. B.: The effects of large doses of Benze-drine Sulphate on the albino rat: Functional and tissue changes, Ann. Int. Med., 10: 1874–88, 1937.
58. EHTISHAMUDDIN, M.: Tranylcypromine, Lancet, ii: 1015, 1963.
58a. ELLIOTT, H. W., TOLBERT, B. M., ADLER, T. K., & ANDERSON, H. H.: Excre-tion of Carbon-14 by man after administration of morphine-N-methyl-C¹⁴, Proc. Soc. Exper. Biol. & Med., 85: 77–81, 1954.
59. EVANS, J.: Psychosis and addiction to phenmetrazine (Preludin), Lancet, ii: 152–5, 1959.
60. FEDELI, M., & LUMIA, V.: Avvelenamento acuto da amfetamina, Farmaco, 10: 19–23, 1955.
61. FERRERO, R. G. A.: Toxicomanías por drogas sicoestimulantes, Semana méd., 117: 1604–5, 1960.
62. FINCH, J. W.: The overweight obstetric patient with special reference to the use of Dexedrine Sulfate, J. Oklahoma M.A., 40: 119–22, 1947.
63. FISCHER, E.: An unusual complication resulting from amphetamine sulphate (Benzedrine): A case report, M. J. Australia, 46: 361, 1959.
64. FLEMING, A. S.: Amphetamine drugs, Pub. Health Rep., 75: 49–50, 1960.
65. FLETCHER, T. F.: Acute dextroamphetamine sulfate poisoning: Report of a case in a child, Am. J. Dis. Child, 86: 777–9, 1953.
66. FOX, C.: Slimming tablets (Correspondence), Brit. M. J., i: 1624, 1962.
67. FREYHAN, F. A.: Craving for Benzedrine, Delaware M. J., 21: 151–6, 1949.
68. FRIEDENBERG, S.: Addiction to amphetamine sulfate, J.A.M.A., 114: 956, 1940.
69. GAYRAL, & COMBES: Toxicomanie par phényl-1-amino-2-propane (ortédrine et Maxiton), Toulouse méd., 51: 218–20, 1950.
70. GERICKE, O. L.: Suicide by ingestion of amphetamine sulfate, J.A.M.A., 128: 1098–9, 1945.
71. GERSCOVICH, J.: Intoxicación accidental leve por ingestión de sulfato de Benzedrina en un niño de 27 meses, Semana méd., i: 804–6, 1948.
72. GILLIS, A.: Addiction to amphetamines (Correspondence), Brit. M. J., ii: 188, 1962.
73. GLATT, M. M.: Toxic psychosis caused by Preludin, Brit. M. J., i: 460–1, 1957.
74. GOLDSMITH, W. N.: Benzedrine eruption, Proc. Roy. Soc. Med., 32: 269, 1939.
75. GRAHN, H. V.: Amphetamine addiction and habituation, Am. Pract., 9: 387–9, 1958.
76. GRANTHAM, H., MARTIN, C. A., & ROULEAU, Y.: Syndromes psychiatriques consécutifs à l'emploi des amphétamines, Laval méd., 33: 85–9, 1962.
77. GREENWOOD, R., & PEACHEY, R. S.: Acute amphetamine poisoning: An

177

account of 3 cases, Brit. M. J., i: **742–4**, 1957.
78. GREVING, H.: Psychopathologische und koerperliche Vorgaenge bei jahre-langem Pervitinmissbrauch, Nervenarzt, **14**: 395–405, 1941.
79. GULLAT, R.: Acute methamphetamine poisoning in a child, Southern M. J., **50**: 1068, 1957.
80. GUTTMANN, E.: Discussion on Benzedrine: Uses and abuses, Proc. Roy. Soc. Med., **32**: 388–91, 1939.
81. HAGENAU, J., & AUBRUN, W.: Intoxication chronique par le sulfate de Benzédrine, Rev. neurol., **79**: 129–30, 1947.
82. HAHNE, L. J.: Addiction to amphetamine (Benzedrine) sulfate, J.A.M.A., **115**: 1568, 1940.
83. HAMMOND, R. C.: Problems arising from prescribing trends, Canad. M. A. J., **91**: 135, 1964.
84. HAMMOND, R. C.: Personal communication.
85. HAMPTON, W. H.: Observed psychiatric reactions following use of amphetamine and amphetamine-like substances, Bull. New York Acad. Med., **37**: 167–75, 1961.
86. HARA, Z., KOGUCHI, G., ANDO, Z., HAGIWARA, Y., MIYASHITA, T., KONNO, O., SHIRAKI, H., SERIZAWA, Y., SATAKE, S., & KURITA, H.: Investigation of chronic amphetamine toxicosis (in Japanese), J. Jap. Soc. Int. Med., **43**: 663–4, 1954.
87. HARDER, A.: Ueber Weckamin-Psychosen, Schweiz. med. Wchnschr., **77**: 982–5, 1947.
88. HART, H. M.: Amphetamine sulfate preparations (correspondence), J.A.M.A., **140**: 1070, 1949.
89. HARTMANN, K.: Pervitin-Halluzinose, Psychiat. Neurol. (Basel), **106**: 101–13, 1942.
90. HARVEY, J. K., TODD, C. W., & HOWARD, J. W.: Fatality associated with Benzedrine ingestion: A case report, Delaware M. J., **21**: 111–15, 1949.
91. HAY, G.: Severe reaction to monoamino-oxidase inhibitor in a dexampheta-mine addict, Lancet, ii: 665, 1962.
92. HERMAN, M., & NAGLER, S. H.: Psychoses due to amphetamine, J. Nerv. & Ment. Dis., **120**: 268–72, 1954.
93. HERNANDEZ, R., & DALMAU, C. J.: The psychodynamics of schizophrenic reactions in Benzedrine poisoning, Bol. Asoc. méd. Puerto Rico, **40**: 163–8, 1948.
94. HERTZOG, A. J., KALSTROM, A. E., & BECHTEL, M. J.: Accidental amphetamine sulfate poisoning, J.A.M.A., **121**: 256–7, 1943.
95. HEUYER, G., & LEBOVICI, S.: Une nouvelle toxicomanie: le Maxiton. A propos de deux observations, Ann. Médico-psychol., **108**: 353–4, 1950.
96. HOFFER, A., & OSMOND, H.: The adrenochrome model and schizophrenia, J. Nerv. & Ment. Dis., **128**: 18–35, 1959.
97. HOPKIN, B., & JONES, C. M.: Dextroamphetamine poisoning (Correspon-dence), Brit. M. J., i: 1044, 1956.
98. HOWARD, C.: Amphetamine in pulmonary tuberculosis (Correspondence), Lancet, i: 44–5, 1947.
98a. ISBELL, H., & FRASER, H. F.: Addiction to analgesics and barbiturates, Pharmacol. Rev., **2**: 355–97, 1950.
98b. ISBELL, H., & WHITE, W. M.: Clinical characteristics of addictions, Am. J. Med., **14**: 558–65, 1953.
99. ISSEKUTZ, B.: Vergiftung durch Pervitin, Arch. Toxicol., **10**: 85–8, 1939.
100. IVY, A. C., & KRASNO, L. R.: Amphetamine (Benzedrine) sulfate: A review of its pharmacology, War Med., **1**: 15–42, 1941.
101. IVY, A. C., & GOETZL, F. R.: d-Desoxyephedrine: A review, War Med., **3**: 60–77, 1943.
102. JACOBSEN, E.: Studies on the subjective effects of the cephalotropic amines

178

in man. II. A comparison between beta-phenylisopropylamine sulphate and a series of other amine salts, Acta med. Scandinav., **100**: 188–202, 1939.

103. JACOBSEN, E., & WOLLSTEIN, A.: Studies on the subjective effects of the cephalotropic amines in man. I. Beta-phenylisopropyl amine sulphate, Acta med. Scandinav., **100**: 159–87, 1939.

104. JORDAN, S. C., & HAMPSON, F.: Amphetamine poisoning associated with hyperpyrexia, Brit. M. J., ii: 844, 1960.

105. JULIEN, R. G., & VINCENDEAU, J.: Hétérochromie de Fuchs, glaucome et sympathomimétiques, Bull. Soc. opht. France, 187–8, 1956.

106. KAGA, T.: Statistics of toxicoses due to stimulants in the Musashino Mental Hospital (in Japanese), Psychiat. Neurol. Jap., **55**: 891, 1954.

107. KAUVAR, S. S., HENSCHEL, E. J., & RAVIN, A.: Toxic eruption due to amphetamine sulfate and its analogue dextroamphetamine sulfate, J.A.M.A., **122**: 1073–4, 1943.

108. KEITER, W. E., & ARNOLD, J. H.: Acute Dexedrine intoxication in children, Arch. Pediat., **72**: 126–8, 1955.

108a. KEY, B. J.: The effects of drugs in relation to the afferent collateral system of the brain stem, Electroencephalog. & Clin. Neurophysiol., **18**: 670–9, 1965.

108b. KEYSERLINGK, H.: Pervitin, Psychiat. Neurol. Med. Psychol. (Lpz.), **2**: 1–9, 1950.

109. KILOH, L. G., & BRANDON, S.: Habituation and addiction to amphetamines, Brit. M. J., ii: 40–3, 1962.

110. KNAPP, P. H.: Amphetamine and addiction, J. Nerv. & Ment. Dis., **115**: 406–32, 1952.

111. KUENSSBERG, E. V.: Diethylpropion (Correspondence), Brit. M. J., ii: 729–30, 1962.

112. KUENSSBERG, E. V.: Diethylpropion and addiction (Correspondence), Brit. M. J., ii: 1406, 1963.

113. LANCER, K.: Idiosyncrasy to dexamphetamine, Brit. M. J., i: 505, 1961.

114. LANGHAM, S. T.: Dexedrine poisoning, Brit. M. J., ii: 892, 1950.

115. LAURENT, J.-M.: Toxique et toxicomanie peu connus, "le cath," Ann. médico-psychol., **120**: 649–57, 1962.

116. LEAKE, C. D.: The Amphetamines—Their Actions and Uses, Springfield, Charles C. Thomas, 1958.

117. LESSES, M. F., & MYERSON, A.: Benzedrine Sulfate (Correspondence), J.A.M.A., **110**: 1507–8, 1938.

118. LIDDELL, D. W., & WEIL-MALHERBE, H.: The effects of Methedrine and of lysergic acid diethylamide on mental processes and on the blood adrenaline level, J. Neurol. Neurosurg. & Psychiat., **16**: 7–13, 1953.

119. MARLEY, E.: Response to some stimulant and depressant drugs of the central nervous system, J. Ment. Sc., **106**: 76–92, 1960.

120. MARTIMOR, E., NICOLAS-CHARLES, P., & DEREUX, J.: Délires amphétaminiques, considérations physiopathologiques et médico-légales, Ann. médico-psychol., **113**: 353–68, 1955.

121. MASAKI, T.: The amphetamine problem in Japan, W. H. O. Tech. Rep. Ser., **102**: 14–21, 1956.

122. MASON, A.: Fatal reaction associated with tranylcypromine and methylamphetamine, Lancet, i: 1073, 1962.

123. McCANN, K.: Slimming tablets (Correspondence), Brit. M. J., ii: 53, 1962.

124. McCONNELL, W. B.: Addiction to amphetamines (Correspondence), Brit. M. J., ii: 412, 1962.

125. McCONNELL, W. B.: Amphetamine substances in mental illness in Northern Ireland, Brit. J. Psychiat., **109**: 218–24, 1963.

126. McCONNELL, W. B., & McILWAINE, R. J.: Amphetamine substances and mental illness in Northern Ireland, Ulster M. J., **30**: 31–4, 1961.

127. McCORMICK, T. C.: Toxic reactions to the amphetamines, Dis. Nerv. System, 23: 219–24, 1962.
127a. McCORMICK, T. C., & McNEEL, T. W.: Acute psychosis and Ritalin abuse, Texas State J. Med., 59: 99–100, 1963.
128. MITCHELL, H. S., & DENTON, R. L.: Overdosage with Dexedrine, Canad. M. A. J., 62: 594–5, 1950.
129. MODELL, W.: Status and prospect of drugs for overeating, J.A.M.A., 173: 1131–6, 1960.
130. MONROE, R. R., & DRELL, H. J.: Oral use of stimulants obtained from inhalers, J.A.M.A., 135: 909–15, 1947.
131. MYERSON, A.: Addiction to amphetamine (Benzedrine) sulfate, J.A.M.A., 115: 2202, 1940.
132. NANDELSTADH, O. W. VON: On Benzedrine psychoses, Acta psychiat. scandinav., Suppl., 60: 64–65, 1951.
133. NODA, H.: Concerning wake-amine intoxication (in Japanese), Kurume Igakkai Zasshi 13: 294–8, 1950.
134. NORMAN, J., & SHEA, J. T.: Acute hallucinosis as a complication of addiction to amphetamine sulfate, New England J. Med., 233: 270–1, 1945.
135. O'FLANAGAN, P. M., & TAYLOR, R. B.: A case of recurrent psychosis associated with amphetamine addiction, J. Ment. Sc., 96: 1033–6, 1950.
136. ONG, B. H.: Dextroamphetamine poisoning, New England J. Med., 266: 1321–2, 1962.
137. OSWALD, I., & THACORE, V. R.: Amphetamine and phenmetrazine addiction, physiological abnormalities in the abstinence syndrome, Brit. M. J., ii: 427–31, 1963.
138. PARKER, J. M., & HILDEBRAND, N.: Fatal reaction associated with tranylcypromine and methylamphetamine (Correspondence), Lancet, ii, 246, 1962.
139. PATERSON, M. C.: Addiction to drinamyl (Correspondence), Brit. M. J., ii: 684, 1963.
140. PATHY, M. S.: Acute amphetamine poisoning, Brit. M. J., i: 946, 1957.
141. PATUCK, D.: Acute dexamphetamine sulphate poisoning in a child, Brit. M. J., i: 670–1, 1956.
142. PETERSON, B. H., & SOMERVILLE, D. M.: Excessive use of Benzedrine by a psychopath, M. J. Australia, ii: 948–9, 1949.
143. PONTRELLI, E.: Sopra un caso di avvelenamento mortale da solfato di beta-fenilisopropilamina (Simpamina), Gior. clin. med., 23: 591–600, 1942.
144. POTELIAKHOFF, A., & ROUGHTON, B. C.: Two cases of amphetamine poisoning, Brit. M. J., i: 26–7, 1956.
145. POTTIER, C., GEORGELIN, R., & COUEDIC, H.: Psychose hallucinatoire par intoxication amphétaminique, Ann. Médico-psychol., 111: 220–4, 1953.
146. POUS CHAZARO, E.: Los inhaladores de Benzedrina, Gac. méd. México, 71: 563–4, 1941.
147. PRATAP, H. J.: Slimming tablets (Correspondence), Brit. M. J., ii: 53, 1962.
148. PRETORIUS, H. P. J.: Dexedrine Vergiftiging, Twee Gevalle Waarven een Noodlottig, South African M. J., 27: 945–8, 1953.
149. RAPP, R. T.: Dexedrine poisoning in an infant, West Virginia M. J., 49: 184, 1953.
150. RICKMAN, E. E., WILLIAMS, E. Y., & BROWN, R. K.: Acute toxic psychiatric reactions related to amphetamine medication, Med. Ann. D.C. 30: 209–12, 1961.
151. ROEBUCK, B. E.: Diethylpropion and addiction (Correspondence), Brit. M. J., ii: 936, 1963.
152. ROECKER, R. D., & LANE, M.: Stupor from dextroamphetamine-amobarbital and monoamino oxidase inhibitor, Phenelzine. J. M. Soc. New Jersey, 58: 47–9, 1961.

180

153. Röhl, K.: Zur Frage der Erzeugung von Süchten durch 1-phenyl-2-methyl-aminopropanhydrochlorid, Arzneimittel-Forsch., 6: 402–6, 1956.
154. Rosen, A., & Oberman, I. J.: Addiction to phenmetrazine hydrochloride and its psychiatric implications, J. Am. Osteopath. A., 59: 722–6, 1960.
155. Rosenbaum, H. A.: Amphetamine sulfate poisoning in a child of twenty months, J.A.M.A., 122: 1011, 1943.
156. Ruiz Ogara, C.: Psicosis desencadenada por choque amphetamínico, Rev. españ. oto-neuro-oftal., 13: 318–23, 1954.
157. Sano, I., & Nagasaka: Ueber chronische Weckaminsucht in Japan, Fortschr. Neurol. Psychiat., 24: 391–4, 1956.
158. Schinko, H., & Solms, W.: Eine Psychose bei Adipexsuechtigkeit, Wien. Ztschr. Nervenh., 9: 290–301, 1954.
159. Schneck, J. M.: Benzedrine psychosis: Report of a case, Mil. Surgeon, 102: 60–1, 1948.
160. Schremly, J. A., & Solomon, P.: Drug abuse and addiction: Reporting in a general hospital, J.A.M.A., 189: 512–14, 1964.
161. Schulz, E.: Intoxikationspsychosen bei Prostituierten nach Preludinmissbrauch, Oeffentlicher Gesundheitsdienst (Stuttgart), 23: 287–91, 1961.
162. Scott, P. D.: Amphetamine and delinquency (Correspondence), Lancet, ii: 534–5, 1964.
163. Seager, C. P., & Foster, A. R.: Addiction to unrestricted drugs, Brit. M. J., ii: 950–2, 1958.
164. Shanson, B.: Amphetamine poisoning, Brit. M. J., i: 576, 1956.
165. Shorvon, H. J.: Use of Benzedrine Sulphate by psychopaths: The problem of addiction, Brit. M. J., ii: 285–6, 1945.
166. Sicé, J.: General Pharmacology, p. 393. Philadelphia & London, W. B. Saunders Co., 1962.
167. Silverman, M.: Subacute delirious state due to Preludin addiction, Brit. M. J., i: 696–7, 1959.
168. Simpson, W. S.: Toxic psychosis: A complication of overdosage of anti-obesity drugs, J. Kansas M. Soc., 58: 524–7, 1957.
169. Smith, L. C.: Collapse with death following the use of amphetamine sulfate, J.A.M.A., 113: 1022–3, 1939.
170. Staehelin, J. E.: Pervitin-Psychose, Ztschr. ges. Neurol. Psychiat., 173: 598–620, 1941.
171. Stungo, E.: "Addiction" to anorexigenic drugs, Med. Press, 246: 76–80, 1961.
172. Stungo, E.: Addiction to amphetamines (Correspondence), Brit. M. J., ii: 339, 1962.
173. Tatetsu, S.: Pervitin-Psychosen, Folia psychiat. neurol. Jap., Suppl., 6: 25–33, 1960.
174. Temkin, L.: Reaction to amphetamine, Lancet, i: 669, 1953.
175. Tolentino, I.: Considerazioni psicopatologiche e cliniche su due casi di Tossicomania e psicosi da derivati fenilpropilaminici, Riv. neurol., 28: 81–90, 1958.
176. Tolentino, I., & D'Avossa, B.: Psicosi da amine simpaticomimetiche, Arch. Psicol. Neurol., 18: 127–169, 1957.
177. Tonks, C. M., & Livingston, D.: Monoaminooxidase inhibitors (Correspondence), Lancet, i: 1323–4, 1963.
178. Trethowan, W. H.: Addiction to amphetamines (Correspondence), Brit. M. J., ii: 188, 1962.
179. Trouton, D., & Eysenck, H. J.: In Handbook of Abnormal Psychology, ed. by H. J. Eysenck. New York, Basic Books, Inc., 1961.
180. Vademecum International, Montreal, J. Morgan Jones Publications Ltd., Products Information, p. 76, 1965.

181. Vademecum International, Montreal, J. Morgan Jones Publications Ltd., Products Information, p. 239, 1965.
182. VIDAL FREYRE, A.: Intoxicación accidental por la ingestión de Sulfato de Benzedrina en un niño de 25 meses, Día méd., 19: 840, 842, 1947.
183. VILL, H.: Stark verlaengerte QT-Zeit im EKG bei akuter Pervitinvergiftung, Cardiologia, 34: 190–6, 1959.
184. WALKER, P. G. M. G.: Diagnosis of amphetamine addiction (Correspondence), Brit. M. J., i: 384–5, 1965.
185. WALLIS, G. G.: Amphetamine psychosis, Brit. M. J., i: 1121, 1957.
186. WALLIS, G. G., McHARG, J. F., & SCOTT, O. C. A.: Acute psychosis caused by dextro-amphetamine, Brit. M. J., ii: 1394, 1949.
187. WALSH, J.: Psychotoxic drugs: Dodd bill passes Senate, comes to rest in the House; critics are sharpening their knives, Science, 145: 1418–20, 1964.
188. WATTS, C. A. H.: Amphetamine poisoning, Brit. M. J., i: 234–5, 1956.
189. WAUD, S. P.: The effects of toxic doses of benzyl methyl carbinamine (Benzedrine) in man, J.A.M.A., 110: 206–7, 1938.
189a. WAY, E. L., SIGNOROTTI, B. T., MARCH, C. H., & PENG, C.-T.: Studies on the urinary, fecal and biliary excretion of dl-methadone by countercurrent distribution, J. Pharmacol. & Exper. Therap., 101: 249–58, 1951.
190. WEISS, B., & LATIES, V. G.: Enhancement of human performance by caffeine and the amphetamines, Pharmacol. Rev., 14: 1–36, 1962.
191. WELSH, A. L.: Side Effects of Anti-Obesity Drugs, Springfield, Charles C. Thomas, 1962.
192. W.H.O.: Expert Committee on Addiction-producing Drugs: Definition of addiction-forming and habit-forming drugs, W.H.O. Techn. Rep. Ser., 21: 6–7, 1950.
193. W.H.O.: Expert Committee on Addiction-producing Drugs: Definitions formulated during the second session of the committee, W.H.O. Techn. Rep. Ser., 57: 9–10, 1952.
194. W.H.O.: Expert Committee on Addiction-producing Drugs: Definition of habit-forming drugs, W.H.O. Techn. Rep. Ser., 116: 9–10, 1957.
195. W.H.O.: Expert Committee on Addiction-producing Drugs: Terminology in regard to drug abuse, W.H.O. Techn. Rep. Ser., 273: 9–10, 1964.
196. W.H.O.: Expert Committee on Addiction-producing Drugs: Khat (Catha edulis), W.H.O. Techn. Rep. Ser., 273: 10, 1964.
197. WIKLER, A.: In The Relations of Psychiatry to Pharmacology. Baltimore, Williams & Wilkins, Co., 1957.
198. WILKIE, D.: Addiction to amphetamines (Correspondence), Brit. M. J., ii: 730, 1962.
199. WILSON, C. W. M., & BEACON, S.: An investigation into the habituating properties of an amphetamine-barbiturate mixture, Brit. J. Addict., 60: 81–92, 1964.
200. YOUNG, D., & SCOVILLE, W. B.: Paranoid psychosis in narcolepsy and the possible danger of Benzedrine treatment, Med. Clin. N. America, 22: 637–45, 1938.
201. YOUNG, G. G., SIMSON, C. B., & FROHMAN, C. A.: Clinical and biochemical studies of an amphetamine withdrawal psychosis, J. Nerv. & Ment. Dis., 132: 234–8, 1961.
202. ZONDEK, L.: Amphetamine abuse and its relation to other drug addictions, Psychiat. Neurol. (Basel), 135: 227–46, 1958.

Index

102–7, 142–4, 149, 160; and mental background of patients, 39; psychosis from, 31–2, 34–5, 37–76, 162, 164–6, 172; reasons given for taking drugs, 20, 64, 66, 169–72; relapses after withdrawal, 49, 50–3, 61–2, 156, 173; schizophrenia coexisting with, 56; social significance of, 133–7; symptoms of, 104, 163–7; with toxic effects, 34–6; in United Kingdom, 107–14, 141–2, 149, 166; in United States, 114–17, 168–9; without ill effects, 32–4; without psychosis development, 88–9. *See also* Dependence on drugs; Withdrawal of drugs

Cocaine, 153, 155
Coma, in intoxication, 23
Compulsion to take drugs, 78, 94, 96
Confusion states, after withdrawal, 49
Connell's description of amphetamine psychosis, 39–41
Criminal behavior, and drug use, 94, 107, 171
Czechoslovakia, phenmetrazine abuse in, 141

DEFINITIONS: of addiction, 78, 80, 86; of drug dependence, 79, 80, 86; of habituation, 78, 80, 86
Delusions of persecution, 20, 23, 40, 48, 50–3, 54, 55, 162, 165–6
Dependence on drugs: abstinence syndrome, 78, 86, 95, 100, 150–1, 164; amphetamine-like drugs, 122–32; amphetamines, 77–121; behavior changes with, 5, 94; in Canada, 117–19; case histories of, 90–3; characteristics of, 79, 86, 87–102; comparisons with narcotics, 100, 150, 156, 171; definitions of, 79, 80, 86, 149; and excretion rate of drugs, 100–1, 151; experimental studies of, 144, 151; incidence of abuse, 35, 101; in Japan, 102–7, 142–4, 149, 160; pharmacological factors in, 98, 142, 148–57; physical effects of, 95, 96–7; psychological factors in, 98, 151–2, 155–6, 169–72; and sleep pattern, 96–7, 150; social significance of, 133–7; studies with

Drinamyl, 97–9; and substitution of drugs, 101; in teenagers, 103, 110–11, 113, 117; treatment of, 144, 156, 173; in United Kingdom, 107–14; in United States, 114–17; without psychosis development, 88–9. *See also* Withdrawal of drugs
Depression: as abstinence reaction, 60, 95, 100, 150, 163–4; from amphetamines, 48, 54, 55; treatment of, 6, 36, 66
Dermatitis, from amphetamines, 35, 95
Diethylpropion: abuse of, 107, 118, 129–32; action of, 68, 110; structural formula of, 4
Dosage: and acute intoxication in children, 7–8, 9; in chronic amphetamine abuse, 39–40, 42–47, 67–8, 86, 104, 149; intravenous, 141, 145, 153–5, 167–8; in phenmetrazine abuse, 124; without psychosis development, 88–9; and toxic state in adults, 17–19, 20, 22, 26
Drinamyl: abuse of, 110–11; studies with, 97–9
Drugs used with amphetamines, 11, 12, 17–19, 26, 28, 35, 42–7, 55–6, 60, 64, 69, 88–9, 95, 154, 169
Drugs used with phenmetrazine, 124
Duration of use of drugs, 154; in amphetamine psychosis, 42–7, 69; in phenmetrazine abuse, 124; without psychosis development, 88–9
Dyspnea, in intoxication, 23

ENGLAND. *See* United Kingdom
Ephedrine: in illicit samples, 153; structural formula of, 4
Epidemic drug use, 102–3, 142–4, 149, 160, 168–9
Epinephrine: metabolism of, in schizophrenia, 73; structural formula of, 4
Euphoria, 5, 11, 111, 135, 152, 161–2, 168, 173
Excitation, drug-induced, 8, 11, 23, 48, 167
Excretion of amphetamines, 100–1; in urine, 40, 55, 75, 113, 137, 150–1

FATALITIES FROM DRUGS: in adults, 23,

Methamphetamine: addiction to, 81; effects of, 153; intravenous use of, 141, 144, 149, 153, 166; psychosis from, 105; structural formula of, 4. *See also* "Speed"

Methylphenidate, abuse of, 128

Mexico, amphetamine poisoning in, 20

Mono-amine oxidase inhibitors, toxicity with amphetamines, 28

Morocco, amphetamine poisoning in, 20

Morphine, 101, 151

Motor excitation, from drugs, 8, 11

Mydriasis: from amphetamines, 4, 8, 23, 59; from drugs, 161

NALORPHINE, 151

Narcolepsy, treatment of, 5, 31, 33, 55, 143

Needle dependence, 155–6

North America, amphetamine abuse in, 141–4, 149, 160–73

Northern Ireland, amphetamine abuse in, 35–6, 109–10

Norway, amphetamine psychosis in, 38, 74

OBESITY, control of, 5, 31, 59, 64, 66, 122, 143

Occupation, and amphetamine psychosis, 64, 65–6

Opiates, dependence on, 100–1, 150, 156, 171–2

PANHEMOCYTOPENIA, 35

Paraldehyde, for amphetamine intoxication, 11

Paranoid symptomatology. *See* Persecutory ideas

Parkinsonism, postencephalitic, treatment of, 34

Pathogenesis of amphetamine psychosis, 72–3

Persecutory ideas, 20, 23, 40, 48, 50–53, 54, 55, 162, 165–6

Personality: and amphetamine psychosis, 70, 164–5; amphetamines affecting, 94; and chronic use of amphetamines, 39, 169–72

Phenmetrazine: abuse of, 107, 118, 123–8, 141, 143, 153; action of, 68, 122; addiction to, 80, 123–8; effects of, 144; psychosis from, 124, 126; structural formula of, 4; withdrawal of, 86

Philoponism, 102

Physical condition of patients, in psychotic episode, 59

Physical effects of dependence on drugs, 95, 96–7, 164, 166

Pipradrol, effects of, 122

Placebos, effects of, 98

Postural function, enhancement of, 59

Preludin. *See* Phenmetrazine

Pseudo-amphetamine psychosis, 56

Psychosis from amphetamines, 31–2, 34–5, 37–76, 162, 164–6, 172; age factors in, 63; case histories of, 57–9; clinical characteristics of, 41–75; described by Connell, 39–41; diagnosis of, 40–1, 55; and dosage range, 67–8; duration of, 40; effects of withdrawal, 60–1; follow-up studies, 61–3; incidence of, 37–8, 41, 74–5; in Japan, 103, 105; and marital status, 65; and mental background of patients, 69–74, 164–5; mental condition during psychotic episode, 41–59, 165; occupational factors in, 64, 65–6; pathogenesis of, 72–3; and physical condition of patients, 59; preparations producing, 67–68; pseudo, 56; sex factors in, 63–5; symptoms of, 37, 40, 48, 50–3, 54–5; and tolerance to toxic effects, 68, 69; treatment of, 61, 173

Psychotic reactions: in acute amphetamine poisoning, 20, 23, 24–5; from diethlypropion, 129; lack of, with chronic abuse of drugs, 88–9; from methyphenidate, 128; from phenmetrazine, 124, 126; after withdrawal of amphetamines, 49, 54, 60–1

Puerto Rico, amphetamine poisoning in, 16

REASONS, for taking amphetamines, 20, 64, 66, 169–72

Reference, ideas of, 37, 40, 48, 54, 72

Relapses, after withdrawal, 40, 50–3, 61–2, 156, 173

Reporting of drug abuse, 115

Respiratory disturbances, in intoxication, 23

Restlessness, from drugs, 23, 35, 36

Reticular formation, midbrain, 5, 11, 152
Reward system in brain, 152

SCHIZOPHRENIA: adrenaline metabolism in, 73; amphetamines affecting, 72–3, 164–5; co-existing with amphetamine abuse, 56, 164–5; pseudo-amphetamine psychosis, 56
Scotland. *See* United Kingdom
Sedatives. *See* Barbiturates
Self-administered drugs, 20, 64, 66
Sensitivity, to drugs, variations in, 26, 28, 68, 69, 94
Sensory isolation, in treatment of intoxication, 8, 12
Sensory perception, 5
Sex factors: in adult intoxication, 17–19; in amphetamine psychosis, 63–5; in childhood intoxication, 9; in chronic use of amphetamines, 42–7, 88–9; in intravenous use of amphetamines, 154; in phenmetrazine abuse, 124
Sexual activity, in amphetamine users, 71, 163
Side effects of drugs, 23, 27
Skin eruptions, from amphetamines, 35, 95
Sleep pattern, studies of, 96–7
Sleepiness: as abstinence reaction, 94, 95, 100; control of, 5, 8, 27, 35, 59, 95
Spain, amphetamine poisoning in, 20
"Speed": acute effects of, 161–3; composition of, 153–6, 160; dosage, 153–5, 167–8; pattern of use, 141–2, 144, 153–5, 160–73; physical complications of, 142, 156, 160, 163–4, 166; social and cultural factors, 142–4, 162–3, 170–1
Stimulatory effects of amphetamines, 5–6, 11
Stomach lavage, for amphetamine intoxication, 8, 11
Suicidal thoughts: and amphetamine use, 40; as withdrawal symptom, 60
Sweden, phenmetrazine abuse in, 141–4, 149, 153
Switzerland: amphetamine poisoning in, 20; amphetamine psychosis in, 37, 74
Symptoms: of amphetamine intoxication, 7, 8, 10, 20, 23, 24–5, 104; of amphetamine psychosis, 48, 50–3, 54–5, 162, 165–6; of drug dependence, 79, 86, 87–102; sympathomimetic, 95, 161; of withdrawal, 40, 60, 61, 100, 150, 163–4

TACHYCARDIA, from amphetamines, 4, 8, 23, 161
Teenage problems with addiction, 103, 110–11, 113, 117
Tenuate. *See* Diethylpropion
Thyroid extract, with amphetamines, 35, 55
Thyrotoxicosis, simulated, 35
Tobacco, 141
Tolerance: pharmacological factors in, 149–51; to toxic effects of drugs, 26, 28, 68, 69, 94
Toxic effects of drugs, 72
Treatment: of amphetamine dependence, 144, 156, 173; of amphetamine intoxication, 11–12; of amphetamine psychosis, 61
Tremors, from drugs, 59
Truck drivers, amphetamine use by, 116

UNITED KINGDOM: amphetamine abuse in, 107–14, 115; amphetamine poisoning in, 16, 29; amphetamine psychosis in, 37, 38, 74; methamphetamine abuse in, 141–2, 149; phenmetrazine abuse in, 127
United States: amphetamine abuse in, 114–17; amphetamine poisoning in, 14, 16, 29; amphetamine psychosis in, 38, 74; methamphetamine abuse in, 168–9
Urine tests, in chronic amphetamine use, 40, 55, 75, 113, 137

VARIATIONS IN SENSITIVITY TO DRUGS, 26, 28, 68, 69, 94
Vasoconstriction, from drugs, 4
Vomiting, from amphetamines, 36

WAKEFULNESS, 5, 8, 27, 35, 59, 95, 152, 161

Weight reduction, drugs for, 5, 31, 59, 64, 66, 122

Withdrawal of drugs: effects of, 60–1, 78, 82, 85, 86, 95, 100; physical changes in, 96; psychotic reactions after, 49, 54, 60–1; relapses after, 40, 50–3, 61–2, 156, 173; sleep pattern in, 96–7; symptoms in, 40, 60, 100, 150–1, 164